WALKS ON THE BEACH WITH ANGIE

Don Warner

May 2008

Walks on the Beach with Angie

A Father's Story of Love

DON WARNER

with Marly Cornell

NORTH STAR PRESS OF ST. CLOUD, INC.

St. Cloud, Minnesota

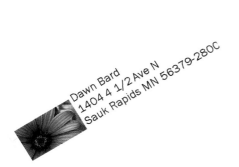

Dawn Bard
1404 4 1/2 Ave N
Sauk Rapids MN 56379-280C

Poem "Footprints in the Sand" by Mary Stevenson. Used with permission.
Poems "Dream" and "Life" by Brian J. Kuhl. Used with permission.
Poem "The Family Room" by Amanda Roy. Used with permission.

Private correspondence of Arthur Roy, Emily Schaefbauer,
Josh Rasmusson. Used with permission.

Scripture quotations taken from the New American Standard Bible®
Copyright © 1960, 1962, 1963, 1968, 1971, 1972, 1973, 1975, 1977,
1995 by The Lockman Foundation. Used with permission.

All photographs collection of Warner family unless otherwise noted.
Cover photo of Angela courtesy of Steve Lucas Photography.

Cover design by Bookwrights.

Some names have been changed to protect privacy.

Library of Congress Control Number: 2008902339

Published by:
North Star Press of St. Cloud, Inc.
PO Box 451
St. Cloud, MN 56302
www.northstarpress.com

Printed in Canada

ISBN 13: 978-0-87839-274-2

Dedication

To my wife Linda—with love and gratitude.

Thank you for being there for Angela
every single day of her life,
and for being the loving and devoted mother
and best friend to our brave and precious child.
You were beautiful together.
Though I cannot fathom the depth of your loss,
we are forever bound by our shared treasure,
heartbreak, and never-ending love.

TABLE OF CONTENTS

FOREWORD

In the early 1960s when I started a clinic at the University of Minnesota Medical School for the treatment of infants with *cystic fibrosis of the pancreas*, the doyen pediatrician in Minneapolis told me, "Warren, let them die. It will be better for everyone."

My reply was, "These are normal babies. Like other children, they catch normal diseases, from which some will die. We just need to improve our preventions and treatments so they can lead normal lives."

Teaching and practicing with that view has made the Minnesota Cystic Fibrosis Center one of the outstanding CF Centers in the world. But we have not yet reached the goal of normal lives for all of our patients.

I met the Warners in 1981 when their baby was diagnosed as having CF. I told Don and Linda that Angie was a normal baby, and with successful preventive treatments, she would grow up to become a normal adult. I cared for Angie for sixteen years. The Warners carried out the best practice of our knowledge perfectly and, so doing, proved my prediction to be true. Angie's full life was one of happiness and many successes, many more than her father has shared in this book.

And yet in 2002 and 2003, we found our knowledge of prevention incomplete. We failed to avert, halt, or reverse the course of the last three months of Angie's life despite the brave and tremendous efforts by Angie and her parents. That part of this book is a strong tale of bravery and sadness. But Don and Linda's plans to brighten the future for older surviving CF patients, through the Angela Warner Foundation, inspires us to do more to help make those adult lives as normal and free of CF problems as possible.

A new part of my research has been stimulated by Don Warner's book; my research will now include the review of thirty-five years of computerized medical records of our CF patients to discover the little things we doctors may have passed over because these details appeared too minor to fuss about at the time. Perhaps, making such a discovery will prevent a future disaster from happening.

We have reason to look forward with hope to the future, for as of January 1, 2008, at the Minnesota Cystic Fibrosis Center there are sixty-nine CF patients over age forty with an average age of forty-eight years. In another ten years, I hope we can write that the Minnesota CF Center has sixty-nine patients over age fifty, average age fifty-eight years, and that we have prevented another outcome from occurring like Angie's last months.

Warren J. Warwick, MD
Professor of Pediatrics
First Annalisa Marzotto Professor for Cystic Fibrosis Patient Care
University of Minnesota Medical School

INTRODUCTION

How unpredictable and uncharted the course of life can be, despite the best-laid plans . . .

While growing up in Princeton, a small town in central Minnesota, I made plans to finish college, find that "good" job, get married and have children—in that order. My unwavering commitment to those goals broke up my high school romance; I wanted to finish my college degree before marriage.

By "good" job, I meant one that paid better than average—the average in our town anyway, and one that didn't involve too much physical labor. I trimmed trees and baled hay before I was sixteen and hated both. Though my family was middle class, my mother struggled to make ends meet after the death of my father.

The insecurity our family experienced during that time instilled in me the strong commitment to achieve security in my own life.

My mother was one of eleven children and her family was poor during and after the Depression. She went to live with another family for a while when her father died. Mom had a high school degree but many of her siblings only reached eighth grade before having to work on the farm. My mother was determined that her children would be well educated, in spite of our financial challenges.

Though I may have inherited my mother's determination, I was much more like my father. He was smart and successful but still liked to have a good time. School was easy for me; I was an A student and scholarship recipient. My friends were fun-loving partiers. I credit the owner of the grocery store where I worked as a teenager for saving me from becoming a kid who partied too much. He taught me that hard work and honesty were required to succeed, no matter how smart you might be.

I moved to Minneapolis to attend the University of Minnesota. I joined a business fraternity, was president of the student body of the Carlson School of Management and received the "Outstanding Business Student of the Year" award.

Phase one of my life's plan was complete.

Right after graduation, I entered the financial planning business with a pioneering firm in St. Paul. The industry was in its infancy and opportunities for success were unlimited. Within a year, another new associate in the firm and I formed a business partnership.

By age twenty-three, phase two of my plan was underway.

I met Linda Kuhl after the Torchlight Parade in downtown Minneapolis the same year. She was sitting in a bar with other members of the parade planning committee. I was attracted to her blonde hair and big smile. Everything else looked great, too. I sent over some popcorn. She smiled, so I joined her. She was a lot of fun and we had a good time together.

I had no specifically defined ideas about what I was looking for in a life partner, but Linda and I shared core values: commitment to family, authenticity, doing for others, and trying to be good people but recognizing that nobody is perfect. Linda was private and content with day-to-day routine, whereas my goal-oriented and competitive we-can-sleep-later nature drove me to fit as much as possible into each day. Our differences were complementary and mutually respected. Linda was a sweet, fun-loving partner.

Phase three was in place when we married in 1978 and moved to the suburbs. Everything in my life was going perfectly according to plan.

By 1980, my business was doing well, and Linda and I were happy together, enjoying life, and ready to start our family. One thing I had not planned and could not have anticipated was the added dimension and depth of love I would feel when our daughter, Angela, was born. I could not have imagined how one tiny person could impact my life so and provide a magnitude of purpose and mission I would have entirely missed by only pursuing my own limited vision of a "life plan."

Then, *WHAM!* My "best laid plans" took an unexpected detour.

Part One

THE WATCH
BEGINS

March 11, 1981, was an unseasonably warm day in the Twin Cities. Linda woke me early that morning to tell me, "It's time." After a pregnancy my wife described as "a breeze," we were about to welcome our first child into the world. But our baby had flipped around into a breech position, requiring a caesarean section delivery. Though I had joined Linda for the pregnancy classes so I could be in the delivery room, special training was required for clearance in the event of a C-section. I was relegated to the fathers' waiting room at Fairview Southdale Hospital in Edina. I tried to read as I waited alone for word of the arrival of our baby. Linda and I had been so excited for this day to come; because we didn't know who was coming we had chosen both a boy's and a girl's name. We had talked about how this new little person was going to assuredly change our lives.

3

Within an hour I was told my wife and our beautiful seven-pound, eight-ounce baby girl were both fine. While Linda was still in the recovery room, a nurse brought Angela Brooke Warner in to meet her father for the first time. She was less than one hour old, wrapped in white blankets. I sat on the couch in the parents' waiting room for the next forty minutes, holding her close. How perfect she was, so content and peaceful as I looked into her bright eyes. I spoke to her softly, telling Angela how much I loved her—that I would always take care of her.

I thought I understood the responsibility of fatherhood prior to that day, but when I looked into the sparkling eyes of this tiny infant, so helpless and dependent, the reality of such awesome love and deep commitment overwhelmed me. I began to cry as she looked back at me. I kissed her soft cheeks again and again. I cannot recall another time in my life when I felt such enormous unbounded joy.

Linda had only seen Angela briefly in the operating room right after surgery. But shortly we were together in Linda's room, marveling at the blessing of our beautiful, healthy baby girl. We could not have imagined how connected we were to become to this child. She'd be the love of our lives, our only child—a future decision not contemplated that day.

The rest of that first day of Angela's life was busy for me. When I wasn't holding her, I made calls to inform family and friends of her arrival or shopped for items Linda needed for her longer-than-planned hospital stay. I bought a stuffed white bunny for Angela. That little bunny acquired the name "Baa Baa" and became Angela's constant bedtime companion. For years to come she fell asleep rubbing its long pink ears to the point where the material became worn and frayed. But on this Wednesday in late winter, Linda and I focused on the precious little miracle before us with her dazzling, attentive eyes and happy spirit.

WITHIN WEEKS AFTER ANGELA CAME HOME, she developed a severe cough that triggered projectile vomiting. She was unable to keep food down. Linda and I worried that our baby wasn't getting sufficient nourishment. Her stomach was upset almost all the time and her sleep was difficult. We carried her around the house virtually all night talking and singing, trying to comfort her. This sometimes worked. For weeks we carried her, walked with her, took her for late-night drives, and comforted her day and night as she struggled with what appeared to be a serious respiratory condition. I was not aware at the time, but the salty taste I noticed when kissing her head was an ominous sign.

The first pediatrician we consulted showed little concern about the cough or Angela's "failure to thrive," as he described her lack of weight gain. He said, "All babies cough. All babies spit up." He had sent us home with a prescription for cough syrup. When the cough medicine did not help, we consulted a second pediatrician. The diagnosis was still inconclusive. Linda and I became increasingly alarmed at Angela's respiratory problems

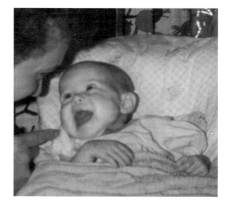

and failure to thrive. Her eyes were hollow and dark. She was becoming weaker, using extra muscles to take each breath. Her condition was worsening.

One morning Angela lay listless and still on our couch. Her eyes were uncharacteristically lifeless; her typically luminous skin looked gray. She wasn't coughing, which might have been interpreted positively except for the other symptoms. At only sixty days old, Angela was telling us that things were "not right." We took her to the emergency room of Minneapolis Children's Hospital.

The doctors immediately shared our concern for Angela. Their initial diagnosis was reflux disease. Food in her stomach was being forced back up into her esophagus and some of this reflux had aspirated into her lungs, causing double pneumonia. The reflux and resulting aspiration, we were told, could be prevented by a minor surgery to correct a flaw in the opening between the stomach and the esophagus. But before surgery could be done, Angela's pneumonia had to clear and her nutritional status needed improvement.

Intravenous therapy immediately provided the needed nutrition, but her respiratory condition worsened. Within one day of her admission, despite IV antibiotics, Angela's right lung collapsed. Several difficult hours followed; her condition was precarious. We almost lost our baby girl.

With more intravenous feedings, Angela was stronger and the pneumonia was gone within a week. We were able to take her home—for a while. The physicians now wanted to take a "wait and see" approach with the stomach surgery.

Linda and I were not convinced that a malfunctioning valve between the stomach and esophagus was enough to explain Angela's symptoms. Her persistent cough seemed too violent for a little baby weighing less than ten pounds. One week after Angela's release from the hospital, with abdominal surgery imminent, we sought the opinion of yet another pediatrician.

After performing several tests, ruling out things like TB, the pediatrician suggested one more test. He said Angela's respiratory condition, along with her digestive problems, could indicate a disease called cystic fibrosis (CF). Neither Linda nor I knew anything about the disease. The doctor assured us Angela's chances of having CF were remote; we should not be concerned until the test could be completed. Her problem might be far less serious. He just wanted to rule out cystic fibrosis first. We were directed to the Cystic Fibrosis Center affiliated with the University of Minnesota for a "sweat" test. Angela's appointment was two days later.

Linda and I both felt some trepidation about being referred to the University of Minnesota Medical Center for our baby's health care. I had spent four years there and graduated from the U, so the physical campus environment was familiar to me. But I had always heard that, if you were very sick in Minnesota, the place to go was either the Mayo Clinic in Rochester or the University of Minnesota Medical Center. Was Angela now one of the *very* sick?

As the three of us went in for the test, Linda and I prayed that our little girl—less than three months old—did not have a dreaded disease that, I sensed, even doctors preferred not to discuss in detail. One of the first questions asked by staff at the CF Center was whether Linda or I had ever noticed that Angela tasted like salt when we kissed her. Of course, by then, we both had noticed. A nurse explained that people with cystic fibrosis have a significantly higher amount of salt in their sweat. The test was to measure the sodium chloride (salt) present in Angela's sweat. Linda and I exchanged glances. Now, mixed with our dread of a serious disease, was also the hope that we were, finally, getting to the bottom of Angela's health problems.

The procedure was painless. Linda held Angela while a colorless, odorless chemical was applied to a small area of skin on her arm. An electrode assisted in stimulating perspiration. A device placed on the skin collected the sweat produced.

We were told to expect a call within a day or so with the results of the laboratory analysis. Of course, we hoped the test would rule out cystic fibrosis, but we were desperate to identify the true source of our daughter's misery and make her healthy. Angela was still having problems keeping food down. Her continual coughing and projectile vomiting made us frantic. We needed answers.

The next afternoon, June 20, 1981, the call came. Linda was told that Angela indeed tested positive for cystic fibrosis; we needed to bring her in to see Dr. Warwick the following day. Linda called me at the office, crying as she told me the news. I headed for home immediately. As I hugged Linda, we vowed to do whatever we could to make our little girl well again. Though we knew nothing of cystic fibrosis, our resolve was firm.

That evening we went to the local library to learn more. The information we found was alarming. Books and magazine articles described the horrors of this incurable disease. Life expectancy for a child with cystic fibrosis was estimated at five to nine years. We were devastated, crushed, shocked. To look at our darling child and think of her dying in less than a short ten years? *Why? Why Angela?*

Our tears flowed; we were so sad and so angry. Several times in the days after Angela's diagnosis, Linda and I felt tempted to close the curtains in the house, sit in the dark, hold our little girl, and just cry. The unfairness of life had held little meaning to me before now. I had been able to overcome every difficulty that I had encountered before in my life. I was sickened to think this fight for Angela might be the only truly important battle I would ever wage—and the predicted grim outcome was apparently already decided.

On our second trip to the Minnesota Cystic Fibrosis Center, we learned more. The Center had the reputation for advancing the life expectancies of their patients to more than twenty years—substantially better than the national average for children with the disease. This was more encouraging than the outdated information we had read in the library.

Linda and I were assured that since we were forced to fight CF with Angela, we were fortunate to be in the Twin Cities. The reputation and success of the CF Center at the university was primarily the result of the dedicated work of one pulmonologist, Warren Warwick, who had been caring for children with cystic fibrosis since 1960. He was devoted to finding a cure for this "child-killer" disease. Linda and I were comforted, knowing he was now Angela's doctor.

Even during our first meeting, we were convinced of Dr. Warwick's commitment to solving the mysteries of cystic fibrosis and to helping our baby. That meeting with him, and each meeting to come, was filled with information and explanations. I sometimes had the feeling he'd prefer to be feverishly at work in a scientific laboratory rather than dealing directly with patients and their families. But his compassion for our child was revealed by an occasional light stroke he gave to Angela's face while he spoke. Tall and somewhat gangly, Dr. Warwick wore heavy-rimmed glasses, and his thinning hair was a bit disheveled. He directed his full attention to Linda and me as he explained details about cystic fibrosis and patiently answered our questions. He referred to diagrams and charts, sketching some anatomical feature if he needed to clarify a point.

We learned that while CF patients face many health issues, the most life threatening are usually the pulmonary complications. A person with CF produces more mucus than normal. The mucus is thick and sticky, so the lungs are not able to clear it out efficiently. If the mucus debris cannot be removed from the lungs, the area will become a breeding ground for bacteria and then pneumonia. In addition, parts of the lungs can become closed off and stop functioning altogether.

My heart ached to think the cough remedy treatments prescribed by the first pediatricians to treat our newborn had been detrimental for her. Cough syrup discouraged Angela's cough rather than helped to clear mucus from her lungs.

The vomiting and stomach problems were also symptoms caused by cystic fibrosis. Angela's "failure to thrive" was the result of her inability to digest her food. Mucus closed the path from the pancreas to the stomach, preventing necessary enzymes from assisting in food digestion. In spite of our best efforts, our baby had been hungry and malnourished. From now on she needed pancreatic enzyme supplements for digestion, and vitamin supplements for adequate nutrition.

Dr. Warwick took pains to assure us that with aggressive and diligent care Angela could live to her thirties or forties. And with the advancements in medicine and genetic research, a cure was not beyond the realm of possibility. He told us about the promising aspects of his own research. Dr. Warwick's words inspired far more hope than the information we'd found on our own. However, to keep our little girl healthy and alive required an extensive and aggressive care program directed by Dr. Warwick and his team. Our lives were about to change in a dramatic way. Only a scheduled, structured life could provide the care Angela required.

ANGELA'S NEW DAILY REGIMEN included two to four aerosol treatments with a drug called Mucomyst, which loosened and thinned the mucus in her lungs. These treatments took fifteen to twenty minutes and were followed by a manual bronchial drainage therapy for thirty more minutes. With cupped hands, we had to pound on our three-month-old daughter in various positions for a half hour each time to help her move the mucus from her lungs.

In addition to the aerosols and bronchial drainage therapies, Angela had to sleep at night in a mist tent. Each evening, we put up sheets that enclosed her bed. A tube inserted through the top blew a soft mist into the tent. The inhaled mist helped to keep the mucus in Angela's lungs moist. Each morning, Angela woke up soaking wet in a wet bed. Then the tent had to be disassembled, the equipment cleaned thoroughly and the sheets washed. The entire routine was repeated each day.

Angela had to ingest multiple daily medications. In addition to nutritional supplements and digestive enzymes, she had to take bronchodilators for help with breathing and general pulmonary function, antibiotics to prevent specific infections, and additional antibiotics as needed. We became regular visitors at our local pharmacy.

Multiple therapies, suctioning, a daunting medication regimen, and cleaning and setting up equipment became our daily routine. Linda carried the entire load if I was away; I covered things when she couldn't be present. And, as every parent knows, caring for a child is a lot of work even without a chronic illness. Schedules, treatments, and quarterly clinic visits became the center of our attention. We became very disciplined.

Linda and I had no hesitation in restructuring our lives. We planned to do whatever was needed to give Angela the best life possible, for as long as possible, hoping and praying always for a cure to be found. Since my financial planning business was doing well, we had decided before Angela was born that Linda would stay home with our child instead of returning to her administrative job in an investment brokerage firm. I was grateful we could afford to make this choice. Linda was a willing and natural caregiver, an ideal mother. An added plus was her comfort with structure and ability to take a methodical approach to accomplishing the tasks needed for Angela's care each day.

Every morning Linda woke Angela to do the first aerosol treatment of the day while I took a shower and ate breakfast. I did the bronchial drainage therapy while Linda prepared medications, cleaned the nebulizer equipment and took care of the mist tent. I placed Angela in nine different positions for three minutes each as I pounded on her with cupped hands. Despite the strong thumping, Angela sometimes slept through the treatments.

A similar schedule was repeated each evening. Angela's eyes were the barometers we could trust. If her eyes were not bright and alert, as they had been at birth, she wasn't feeling well. If she had a cold or other respiratory problem, the therapy regimen was increased, sometimes up to six times a day. Angela fell asleep in my arms while we watched television on our bed at night. Then I carried her to her room, and Linda and I placed her in the mist tent.

With consistent treatments and diligent care, Angela "thrived." She gained weight and her pulmonary function was almost normal. She was a happy baby. Our little angel was doing fine, and her life, while structured, was good. By the time she turned a year old we were ready to celebrate. Her first birthday was a milestone. Linda and I were grateful.

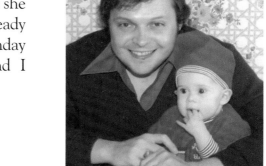

Angela's first Christmas

CHOOSING JOY

Angela was about a year old when special guests came to town—my godparents, Les and Dorothy Jensen, and their white miniature poodle. Dorothy was my father's sister. Les had been like a father to me after my father passed away when I was fourteen. I dearly loved my aunt and uncle. They had driven seventy miles from St. Cloud to meet our baby. We spent most of the afternoon together sitting around the dining room table. Angela and the dog were together on the floor near the table. We talked about Angela's therapies, her prognosis, and the fact that CF was hereditary. We tried together to think of anyone in the family who might have had cystic fibrosis. Dorothy told us about her cousins, two sisters who each had respiratory issues, and both had died very young from pneumonia in the late 1940s or early 1950s. The cause of their ill health was speculation; cystic

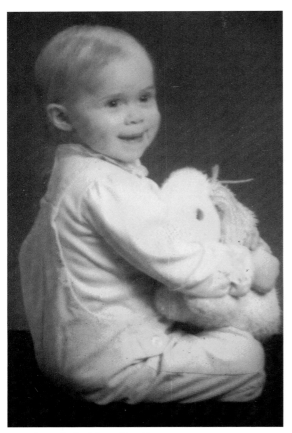

Angela holding Baa Baa

fibrosis had not yet been identified.

We gave each other updates about family events. And, as usual, Les and I talked about business. Les always had jokes and stories to tell. He had the greatest laugh I ever heard—a joyous sound that electrified a room. We were in the middle of our wonderful visit when Les heard Angela's laugh for the first time. The antics of the little poodle playing on the blanket in front of Angela delighted her and she began a hearty and deep laugh, starting as a giggle that escalated and ended with a crescendo howl. Linda and I had been enthralled with that laugh from the start. Les immediately scooped up Angela in his large, strong hands and laughed along with her. What a sight! They had a boisterous laugh together that put everyone in high spirits. Les prompted Angela to laugh once again and their shared hilarity filled the room with happiness.

DESPITE THE ADJUSTMENTS REQUIRED in Angela's first years of life, Linda and I knew how fortunate we were. Angela fully captivated us. Even before she could talk, her attentive eyes expressed so much. She was not going to miss anything. Though such highly structured days required tremendous adaptability on the part of such a young child, Angela was extraordinarily cooperative as we carried out each of her therapies. She accepted structure and the aggressive treatments without complaint, almost as if she understood their importance to her health. Linda and I tried to keep a positive focus on the future. Our goal was for Angela to enjoy her life; we certainly enjoyed her. We worked diligently to keep her lungs clear, make sure she could digest her food, and make her the happiest, most loved little girl possible.

In some ways our job seemed simple enough but, as any family confronting a chronic, life-threatening illness knows, the enormous challenge is in the execution, the details, and the daily grind. We had to face the reality: our little girl would endure a lifetime of medical challenges. We had been told that, for a person with cystic fibrosis, even in the best of cases, breathing is like trying to inhale with a large foot pressing down on your chest. Angela would most likely spend much of her life fighting off pulmonary infections and laboring for each breath. She might not grow and thrive as well as other children.

Though Dr. Warwick predicted Angela's life could extend to her thirties, a great deal of other information we found suggested a far less optimistic outcome. What is a parent to do? How does anyone face a truth that only through a life of dedication and daily intervention could parents help their child reach some future age and, yet, still have to watch their child die? Were we naive to hope a cure could come during Angela's lifetime? Did we have a choice other than to love her and hold onto her for as long as we could have her in our lives? Linda and I knew of no other way but to fight this disease together with all we had, for as long as we were able, without limit or reservation—for Angela.

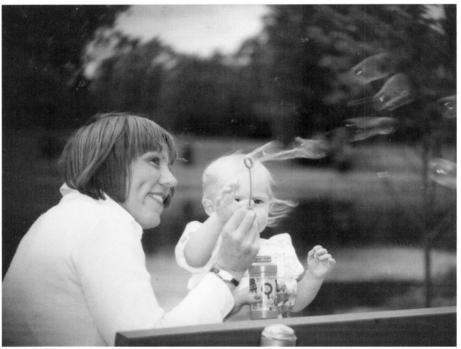

Linda and Angela were beautiful together.

LIKE EVERY CHILD surviving with CF, Angela was a natural-born fighter. From the day of her birth, she fought the disease with her body. From then on, each of us had to fight the disease with our minds and hearts as well. Insurance coverage for certain equip-

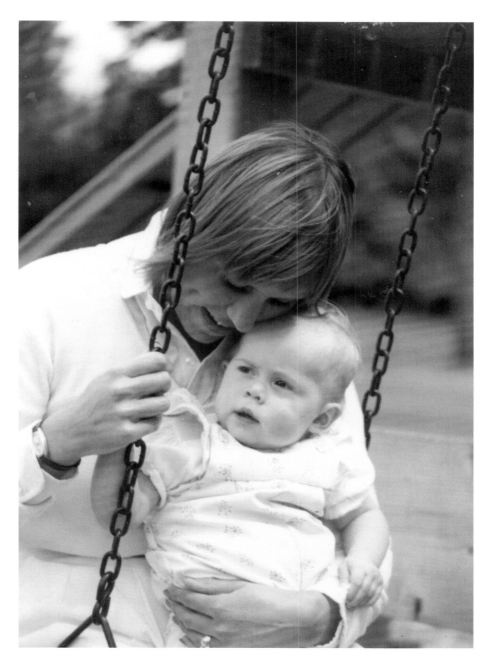

ment and medications was limited or non-existent, so I worked harder to build my financial planning practice to ensure Angela's care was not compromised by financial limitations. I wanted her to have everything she needed to fight cystic fibrosis.

Four times a year, an entire day was spent with evaluations and pulmonary tests at the CF Center. We always went together to clinic visits. Linda and I sincerely felt, and tried to convey to Angela, that she was not alone with cystic fibrosis. We all had CF; we had CF as a family. We placed ourselves side-by-side with her in the battle. But she was the one who had to face this disease directly each day. She was the one who experienced shortness of breath and labored breathing, even on good days.

When Linda and I were asked, by those without a child like Angela, how we felt about having to care for a child with cystic fibrosis, I sometimes sensed an expression of pity toward us. But in our minds, the suffering part of the fight, and any other difficulty involved, was not about Linda or me. Angela was the one who had to live with a disease that would likely rob her of years and experiences. Were our hearts crushed because our little girl had to endure such a disease? *Absolutely.* Did we live in fear from the day of diagnosis forward? *Of course, we did!* Did our challenges and concerns compare in any meaningful way with what Angela had to face? Linda and I didn't think so.

So, AS A FAMILY, we did our best to keep the focus on positive thoughts and activities. We structured our daily lives and our goals to accommodate the health and care of our daughter.

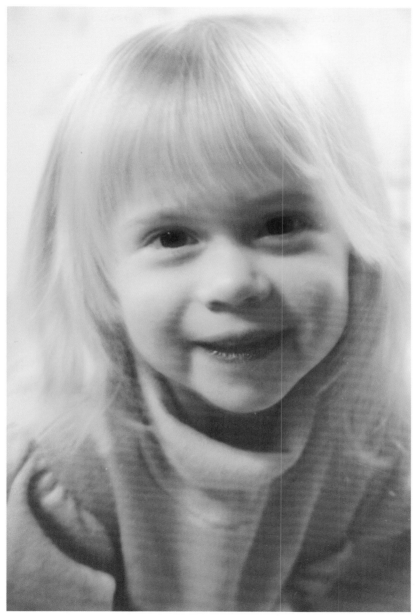

Angela at age three.

OUR FAMILY SPENT THE FIRST THREE YEARS of Angela's life in a double bungalow on two acres of woods in the growing suburb of Eden Prairie. Two years before, my business partner and I developed and built nine double bungalows on a quiet cul-de-sac there. Linda and I decided this place was the ideal home for us to start our family. Angela learned to walk and talk there. Even after we moved to a new home in the fall of 1983, we rented out the double bungalow with a hope to someday give the property to Angela.

The home we moved to in 1983 was also in Eden Prairie. The L-shaped rambler walkout came with a swimming pool in the backyard. Angela was three years old when summer came. I had grown up swimming in lakes around Princeton and wanted my daughter to be comfortable in the water. I came home from work before dinner each day in the summer for "pool time" with Angela. Initially, she was only interested in playing with toys in the shallow end or on the steps into the pool. She instructed me to sit on a step so she could play hairdresser and makeup artist. She worked to make me look "pretty," then dumped a bucket of water on my head so she could start over again. We developed little skits. I pretended to be a "beauty-challenged" character of some sort, coming for help from the "great makeover specialist" Angela. She laughed uproariously at the results. Knowing Linda was watching from the house gave Angela added incentive to work me over.

By the end of the first summer, Angela readily jumped into the pool, went under the water, and floated on her back. By the second summer she swam pretty well. By the third year, at age six,

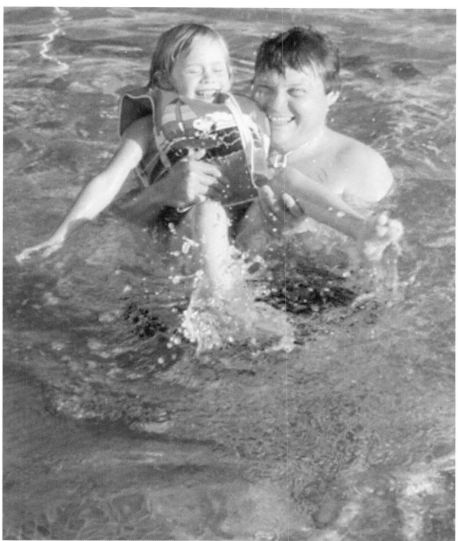

Angela learning to swim

she was swimming "like a fish." She was ready to hit the pool the minute I came home from work. Sometimes, we'd "get crazy" and run and jump into the pool holding hands and screaming at the top of our lungs. We had swim races, played basketball and other games in the pool or just relaxed, rocking or floating together.

Angela was full of energy for winter activities as well. We built snowmen and snow forts in the front yard and sledded down the hill in our backyard. Bundled from head to toe, she could sled for hours. Her cheeks turned red and snow clung to her stocking cap and eyelashes. No matter how cold, Angela never wanted to quit.

LINDA AND ANGELA were inseparable best friends. They played dolls, had "tea" parties, and produced in-home concerts and shows of all kinds. They were beautiful together. Linda introduced Angela to shopping malls and shrewd spending. My girls spent hours searching for "the right item at the right price."

Early on, Linda earned the forever nickname "Mama Bear" and Angela was "Baby Bear." I was, of course, "Papa Bear." But the bear nicknames mostly belonged to the two of them. To me, Angela was "Daddy's Little Princess." Linda had her personal relationship and activities with Angela, and I had mine. However, the three of us were together most of the time, whether traveling, playing, doing therapies or visiting the clinic.

Knowing by now that any other child of ours would face a one-in-four chance of having cystic fibrosis, Linda and I made the difficult decision not to have any other children. Angela's prognosis at that time was too uncertain, and we wanted the ability to fully devote ourselves to her. As we heard about other children and young adults who continued to die from cystic fibrosis, we wondered how many years we'd have with Angela. We made our plans based upon what would be fun for her, packing in as many life experiences as possible. As a result, we had many memorable family celebrations and vacations.

Despite the strong love and wonderful times together during special occasions, and during every ordinary day as well, Linda and I never forgot the cloud that hung over us, the aching concerns about how cystic fibrosis would one day affect Angela. On every birthday, every time any one of us blew out the candles, there was only one wish. No other prayer request was a close second to a cure for cystic fibrosis. Afraid to let our hopes get too high, we prayed for time, enough time for a cure to be found. In the meantime, Angela was our best role model, showing Linda and me how to live a normal life. Her energy and spirit of wonder set the tone.

IN MARCH 1986, Angela was five when we took her on a vacation to San Diego. She played on the beach and visited the San Diego Zoo, Old Town, and SeaWorld. Angela was immediately taken with the dolphins and was full of questions, which I tried to answer. We drove an hour north to a resort called the Surf and Sand in Laguna Beach for several more days. The rooms at the resort were beautiful. I will never forget the look of awe on Angela's face when she threw open the doors leading to the deck and saw nothing but ocean. From our deck we could sometimes see a school of dolphins cruising in the water. Angela shook with excitement until we ran down to the beach to see more.

Walks on the beach became a daily and nightly event for Angela and me on our trip to Laguna. She was fascinated with marine life.

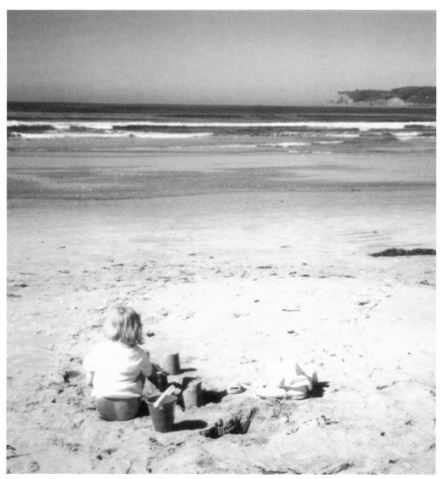

Angela in San Diego

She asked, "Where do dolphins go at night?"

I tried to explain how day and night were not as important a distinction for dolphins or for most ocean dwellers. Angela worried that dolphins might not have enough to eat. I assured her the ocean was filled with edible fish for them. Our conversation moved on to different kinds of fish, and how some live so far down in the deepest parts of the sea that they don't ever see daylight. Angela was wide-eyed, listening to tales of colorful creatures and ocean depths.

"Where do seashells come from?"

I told her that seashells were like leftover armor—grown originally to protect small creatures that were once alive. She collected some and peered closely at them.

At night, Angela and I ran toward the water and back, sometimes misgauging the height and speed of the waves. Soaked and sandy, we usually stopped at the outdoor pool to rinse off under the foot showers before going back to the room to do therapy. We held hands and looked up at the blanket of stars overhead. Angela smiled and said the twinkling lights were so pretty. I agreed with her that the entire sky looked bigger than the view of the stars from our home in the Midwest.

Starting with that trip, Laguna Beach was our family's favorite place in the world. We returned there once or twice every year for more fun and memorable walks on the beach.

IMAGINATION

In the fall of 1986, Angela entered a new stage of life—kindergarten. Angela's first five years had been spent primarily with Linda and me. She had neighborhood friends, some play dates through acquaintances or with her cousins. But she had not been in daycare or preschool. Linda and I were fairly confident that, despite Angela's lack of previous experience with any structured program away from home, she would adapt well to new activities and opportunities. Sure enough, the transition was made successfully with the help of a terrific kindergarten teacher, Pam Olson, whom Angela and Linda called Mrs. O.

Our morning schedule now had to be adapted to fit in Angela's therapy regimen before school. School days began at 5:30 A.M. I ate breakfast and showered while Linda turned off

29

the mist tent, woke Angela and helped her change out of her wet pajamas. Angela sat on the couch in the lower-level family room for the aerosol part of the bronchial drainage therapy. Linda held Angela in her arms and positioned the facemask over her nose and mouth. Angela often fell back to sleep during the twenty-minute aerosol treatment. I took over for thirty minutes of pounding on Angela's chest and back in the nine positions.

At the end of each therapy session, Angela was usually laying over one of my knees with her head hanging down. I scooped her up into my arms and gave her a big hug. By then Linda had prepared Angela's breakfast and set out her twenty to thirty daily pills, including large capsules full of supplemental digestive enzymes that Angela had to take whenever she ate anything. Linda drove her to school and picked her up when school was done. Angela talked on the ride home about whatever happened at school that day and, later, she told me about her day while we did evening therapies together.

Weekend mornings differed only in that we turned off the mist tent and let Angela sleep longer. If she was damp from the mist, Linda or I changed her clothes and let her go back to sleep. However, our morning routine created such an ingrained habit, Angela rarely slept late.

I IMAGINE THAT MOST FAMILIES fighting cystic fibrosis decide early in their child's life whether they will "go public" and be open about their family's struggle against CF or whether they will keep the disease private and try to live every other aspect of life to the

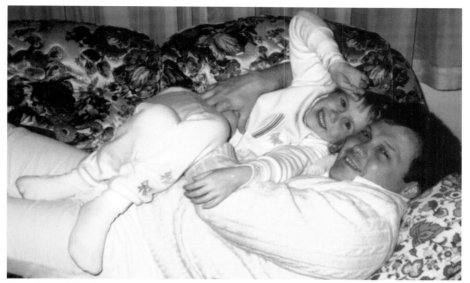

Angela and Dad

outside world as if CF was not present. I could, and still can, see pros and cons to each approach. Perhaps the former can engender more support and create more openness about the disease and the effect of CF on a family. But there is a risk that such a child could become primarily identified with his or her illness or be treated differently than other kids. This issue wasn't a subject we actually discussed or came to a specific decision concerning; rather, our family seemed to be in sync. Outside of the CF Clinic appointments, we did not discuss the ramifications of CF with Angela, and we never discussed her CF with anyone unless necessary. Only family and close friends knew she had cystic fibrosis.

Angela remained cooperative and diligent in doing what was important or recommended for her health, but she did not want her friends or schoolmates to know about her disease. She focused her life and activities elsewhere. Linda and I respected her feelings and did the same. Following her lead, we did not discuss CF openly, even with other family members.

Although none of Angela's classmates knew about her CF, Mrs. O and each subsequent teacher had to be informed about Angela's CF so they understood why she sometimes had to miss school for a clinic appointment and why she might have frequent CF-related illnesses. On the first day of kindergarten, Linda told Mrs. O about Angela's illness to explain about the supplemental digestive enzyme pills she had to swallow with any food she ate, including any snacks.

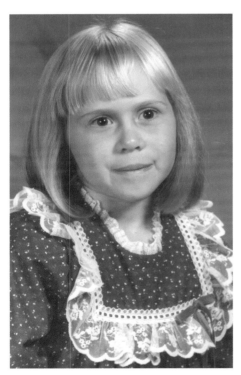

Angela in kindergarten

Mrs. O had a loving heart and responded with emotion when she learned that our little girl had such a terrible disease. She offered to do whatever was necessary and help in any way she could to make sure Angela had a positive kindergarten experience. Angela fell in love with her teacher and looked forward to going to school each day. Mrs. O understood the need for discipline in the classroom, but she also showered her students with loving hugs and kind words.

Pam and Linda became good friends and began the practice

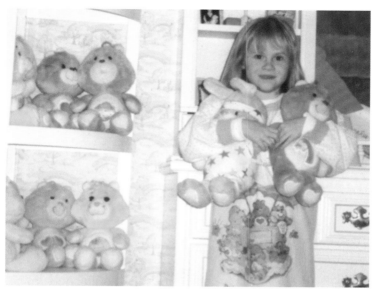

Angela's Care Bears

of getting together for lunch every few months. At the end of kindergarten, Mrs. O gave Angela a white Guardian Angel bear with iridescent, shimmering wings. She said she wanted Angela to have a guardian angel to watch over her as she moved on to first grade and through the years ahead. The bear immediately became Angela's favorite toy, replacing Baa Baa—the little white bunny I had given her the day she was born. Baa Baa was well worn by then. Guardian Angel was an ideal replacement.

ANGELA PARTICIPATED IN EVERY little-girl fad of the day. Along with her stuffed Disney animals and other theme-related toys, like Strawberry Shortcake and Care Bears, she collected dolls. Her first favorite was a beautiful French doll named Ophelié. Though she collected many dolls, she found ways to play with each of them. Her active imagination always impressed me. She held make-believe gymnastics meets, dance contests, or rock concerts. I sometimes observed her playing with other children who eventually sat back to watch as Angela's imagination kicked into full speed. She brought to life pretend settings, people, conversations, and events in elaborate detail. I am certain her imagination partly grew out of her being an only child. Though Linda and I both played often with Angela, she still had plenty of time on her own; she was skilled at entertaining herself and others.

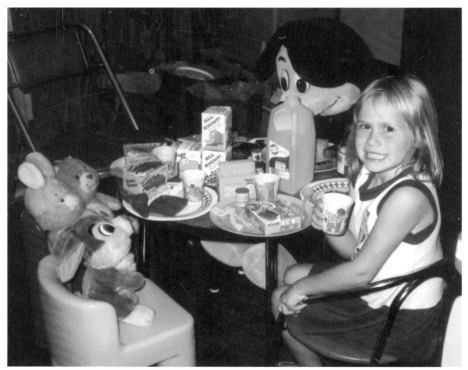

Tea party

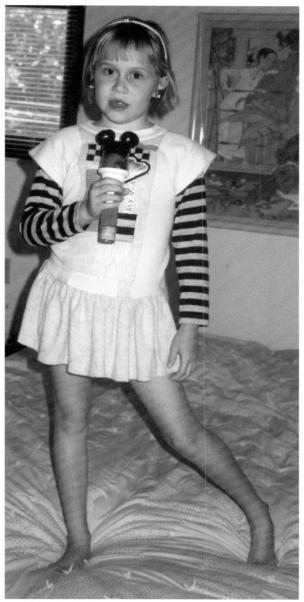

Ladies and Gentlemen . . .

Angela made an audiotape on a snowy winter day when she was six. On the tape, her breathing sounded a little strained due to a cold. She was teaching her bears how to do her therapies. She laid a bear across her lap, the same way I laid Angela across mine, to show the bear all nine treatment positions. She sang, "Doo bop bop, you and me, bop bop. Bop a doo, bop bop. Bop bop bop, bop a doo."

She played with a group of dolls about the size of Barbie dolls that were members of a rock band on a little plastic stage. The dolls had guitars, glittery outfits and wild, ratted hair. Angela had names for each of them. On the tape she introduced the musicians by name, and answered, "Hi," for each of them. She came up with more names than she had dolls: Molly, Jennifer, Ashley, Rachel, Melissa, Roxy, Lauren, Heather, Kelly, Carrie, Tracy, Betsy, Katie, Vicky, Stacy, Kelly [again], Anna, Mickie, Nina, Stephanie, Kia, Tanya, Alicia, Jordan, Angela [of course], Michelle, Bonnie, and Peter [?].

She sang loud, shouting, "We're all together. Come on, Yay!" while the pretend audience jumped up and down. She complimented the musicians, saying, "Good job! You all worked hard on this!" She stopped to sing along to a Whitney Houston tune on the radio and recite short poems such as: "Mommy opened up her drawer and dropped her underwear on the floor!" Her non-stop monologue was punctuated with occasional coughs, as well as screams and shrieks of cascading laughter.

THE FAST-GROWING COMMUNITY of Eden Prairie was building new schools almost annually in those days. Angela went to a different school every two years. She didn't seem to mind the

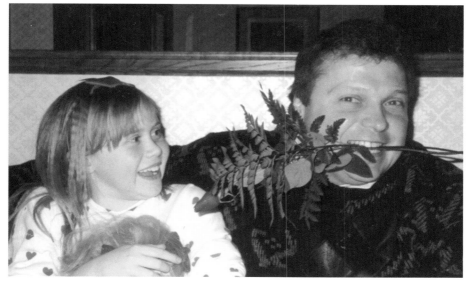

Valentine's Day 1989

changes. She adjusted easily to each new environment and rarely found schoolwork very challenging. She enjoyed going to school but also loved her breaks. One such break occurred in the spring of 1989, when Angela was eight years old. I had a business convention to attend in Oahu, so we were off to Hawaii.

Angela was excited to fly over the ocean. We went to Maui first and stayed in a hotel with a multi-level, enormous pool with waterfalls. We swam, walked on the beach and went to Lahaina in the late afternoon for shopping and dinner. On Oahu we explored Waikiki Beach and other areas around Honolulu. Linda and I had been to Hawaii in 1979 for our first wedding anniversary, but traveling with Angela at age eight was an entirely different kind of fun.

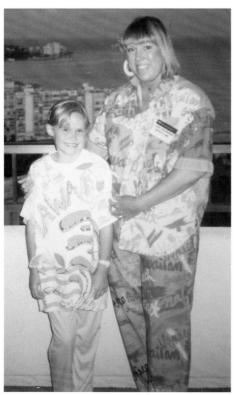

Angela and Linda shopped to find just the right outfits and accessories.

OUR TWICE-A-YEAR TRIPS to Laguna Beach were that way too. I loved being the escort for my two girls. We always went to Disneyland in Anaheim for a day and spent another day at SeaWorld in San Diego. Angela and Linda went to Fashion Island in Newport Beach, and did some "serious" shopping at the South Coast Plaza, Beverly Hills, or La Jolla. My main pleasures were swimming with Angela in the hotel pool, dining together at the end of each day, and our morning and evening walks along the beach.

Angela and I held hands and walked barefoot in the sand at night, looking at stars. We talked about how immense the universe must be, and how small we were in comparison. Our conversations began to include concepts like distance. Angela commented on the brightness of the full moon. When I said that the moon was 240,000 miles away, she was quiet for a moment before asking, "How much further away is that than Hawaii?"

"To get to the moon is as far as one hundred trips to Hawaii."

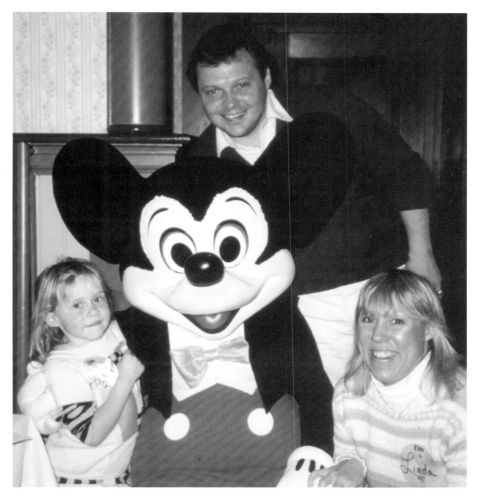

Mickey and the family

I added that the sun was ninety-three million miles from Earth and the stars were much further away. But those distances may have been too abstract for her to grasp at age eight. I could see the moon reflected in her eyes as she stared at the sky and considered these things.

Our family developed some lasting friendships with several people in the Laguna Beach area. We made friends with the owners of a small "foot" jewelry shop, Shelby's, on the Pacific Coast Highway. Roger and Shirley helped Angela select the latest toe rings and ankle bracelets. We stayed in contact with Roger and Shirley throughout the year as well and enjoyed having friends in our favorite vacation area. Angela loved to decorate her feet and ran into the shop first thing to see the new items on each visit. Her enthusiasm for stylish footwear prompted Roger to tell Angela she could have a job working at Shelby's if she ever decided to move to California.

By 1989 THE GENE that caused cystic fibrosis was discovered and the molecular code of the disease was accurately described. This development promised improved screening for cystic fibrosis and more effective therapies. As exciting as the new discovery sounded, there were many more years of research needed before gene therapy could make a difference for current CF patients like Angela. However, thankfully, by the time Angela was ten, another treatment breakthrough made a big difference to Angela, and to me.

Dr. Warwick had been busy perfecting an important medical equipment invention to assist with daily therapies and provide CF patients with much-needed independence. Angela was soon able to do without the manual bronchial drainage therapy in favor of a vest device with an air compressor that pulsated air into the vest at various intervals. The vest was designed to create the same or better results in moving lung secretions than I could manually with all of my pounding on Angela's chest and back in the nine positions.

Dr. Warwick's invention was just in time, because my days doing therapy were soon going to have to end, no matter what. I had developed carpal tunnel syndrome and numbness in both hands from doing multiple daily therapies for more than a decade.

The new high frequency chest compression vest was costly, too new, and possibly too experimental for health insurance companies to be willing to provide reimbursement. Nor would the equipment be widely manufactured or distributed for some time. But we readily agreed to pay the twenty-thousand-dollar price tag to try out the vest. Angela was among the first people with CF to use the new treatment tool. I recalled the words of the CF Center clinician many years earlier, telling Linda and me during our first appointment that we were lucky to live in the Twin Cities if we were fighting cystic fibrosis.

After Angela used the vest for a few weeks, I had some concern about whether this treatment tool was as effective as my aggressive pounding had been. The vibrations created by compressed air didn't seem as strong as my pounding. In addition, Angela was always seated when she used the vest and the lower part of her rib cage wasn't entirely covered. I had turned Angela upside down for some of the therapy positions, which had the added advantage of using gravity to help clear her lungs. Could this vest do as well without any changes in position? I shared my concerns with Dr. Warwick. He cited the research he had been doing and reaffirmed his belief that the vest worked well. I did not understand enough about air compression, so I opted to trust Dr. Warwick and the vest. Besides,

Angela was not about to go back to the pounding. She was quite pleased with the additional independence she had gained with the new equipment. She could now carry out the therapy treatment routine by herself, on her own schedule.

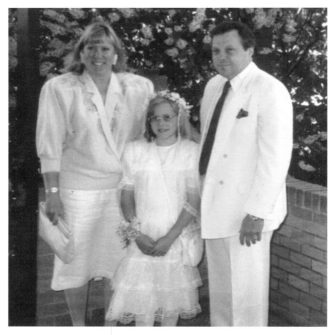

On a gorgeous June day in 1989, Angela received her First Communion at Immaculate Heart of Mary Catholic Church in Minnetonka, Minnesota. Our entire extended family came to our home for a pool party and celebration.

LINDA AND I DECIDED before we were married to worship as Catholics. Linda had grown up in a traditional Catholic family with several uncles and aunts who were nuns and priests. I had grown up Lutheran, but I had developed great respect for the Catholic faith and traditions.

The three of us went to a church in Minnetonka, Minnesota. Angela said nighttime prayers, as Linda and I did privately, but much about our faith was assumed more than discussed within our family. Angela was about eight when we first talked about Heaven. She asked me where my father was "now."

I was fourteen in 1967 when my parents went out to dinner at their favorite restaurant on a Saturday before Christmas. They had spent the afternoon gift shopping. My younger sister Joan and I stayed up late watching television, waiting for them to come home. They usually didn't stay out so late. Shortly after midnight we heard a car in the driveway. Aunt Dorothy and Uncle Les came in the front door with our mother. Mom said nothing as she passed us and went into her bedroom. Les sat down on the arm of the chair where I was sitting, put his arm around me and said, "Something bad has happened."

Dorothy sat talking nearby with her arm around my sister, as Les told me my father had passed away. The original theory was that he'd had a brain hemorrhage, but an autopsy later showed he choked on a piece of meat. Les was a reassuring presence during this loss as he had been only a year and a half before when my eighteen-year-old half-brother, Gary, was killed in a bizarre construction accident.

That hot day in July, a sheriff had come to our house. I had been playing baseball like I did most of the summer. I was standing on our screened-in sleeping porch holding my baseball bat when the sheriff asked if my mother was home. Mom came out on the porch as I leaned on the bat. The sheriff said, "Your son was killed in an accident this afternoon." Gary had been buried in a gravel crusher.

My mother fell to her knees—and my bat fell to the ground. The sheriff helped my mother inside and stayed with her until the pastor from Immanuel Lutheran Church arrived. By evening the house was full of family. My father was out of town, and my other half-brother, Dennis, was away at college. I remember hanging around outside with my cousins, tossing around a baseball. Les and Dorothy arrived the next day.

I had looked up to my brother. Nicknamed "Lefty," Gary loved sports and was on all the local teams. He played first base and pitched. I missed him. Joan and I heard our mother sobbing night after night. I felt so bad for her. Mom had lost her father when she was a child, and lost her first husband to a farm accident when Dennis was three and she was pregnant with Gary. She'd married my father when the boys were still small. But of all my mother's tragic experiences, Gary's death was the one that broke her heart.

Ours was a stoic German family; little was said out loud about what happened to Gary. Death was not a topic of conversation in our home. My father may have been trying to relieve my fears and concerns about my brother when he took me fishing soon after and told me about a near-death experience that happened to him. My father had developed a serious ulcer four years before, requiring him to be rushed into emergency surgery. During that incident, he was clinically dead for several minutes. Dad described being aware of a "wonderful sensation" that began at his feet and coursed throughout his body. That was the only open discussion about death with him that I remember.

A little more than a year later, my father was also gone. During the two or three days before his funeral, I stayed in my room and played Dickie Lee's rendition of Ricky Nelson's "Travelin' Man" over and over on my record player. I thought that no matter how glorious Heaven might be, I was so sad that Gary and my dad had gone to some unknown place, away from anything or anyone familiar.

When Angie asked me about my dad, I downplayed the tragic aspect of my family's past, saying that those things happened long ago. At age eight, Angie accepted my abbreviated version of those losses and the explanation that my father was in Heaven.

ANGELA CONTINUED QUARTERLY VISITS to the CF Center for evaluations, lung function tests, and an examination by Dr. Warwick. She was ten when the conventional wisdom changed regarding mist tents. The way we learned about the change in treatment philosophy was by accident, literally. On a Saturday morning during a light snow, Linda was taking one of her daily six-mile walks when she slipped, fell and broke her ankle. She was not going to be able to do all of her typical daily routines related to Angela's therapies while she healed, especially the mist tent assembly and disassembly each day. At the CF Center a couple of weeks later, Dr. Warwick told us the physicians there had been rethinking the value of the mist tent anyway. He said the benefit of keeping one's airways moist was offset by the risk that a moist environment also created a breeding ground for bacteria.

We didn't want to subject Angela to the mist tent if that form of treatment wasn't good for her, but Linda and I were apprehensive about discontinuing a practice we had been convinced was at least part of the reason Angela had remained healthy for so many years. The original intent of the mist tent made sense to me: by keeping the air in Angela's lungs moist, she could expel mucus more easily.

The same doctor who had once made such a convincing argument for the tent was now saying the mist tent was history. Angela could now sleep in a warm, cozy, dry bed like other children. Linda and I were happy about Angela's newfound comfort and the elimination of the associated daily chores, but we paid close attention to Angie's breathing after the change. Thankfully, her relative good health still remained, without the tent.

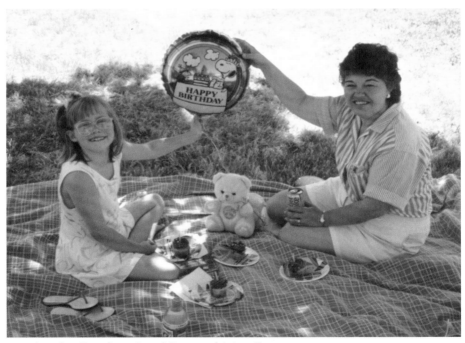

Angela, Guardian Angel Bear, and Mrs. O

Angela underwent annual chest x-rays and a new test that involved inhaling a "nuclear" aerosol followed by x-rays that measured airflow. Through all the tests, Angela's pulmonary function showed very little deterioration and no scarring of the lungs. Once or twice a year she caught a bad cold or developed slight pneumonia. We treated those immediately and aggressively with additional therapies and antibiotics.

Linda and I were well aware that Angela was doing very well compared to most people with CF. Despite the occasional nasty colds that afflicted everyone with cystic fibrosis, she rarely missed a day of school. We *never* took her health for granted.

PART TWO

THE CHEERLEADER

Prior to the 1992 Summer Olympics, the only spectator sports Angela showed interest in were ice skating and gymnastics. She watched videotapes of the competitions again and again during her therapies. Angela had little interest in the sports I was drawn to—baseball, football, and basketball. She had attended occasional games with me over the years but did so only to please me, and then only infrequently. If I tried to force her, we were both miserable. As a father, I had long since resigned myself to living without those hoped-for, regular trips to the ballpark or sports arenas with Angela. My dwindling wish for such a sports bond seemed trivial, a small thing to do without; my daughter brought so much other richness to my life. But then, along came the 1992 NBA Basketball "Olympic Dream Team!"

The 1992 Summer Olympics was the first time America sent a basketball team composed of NBA All Stars. The team was made up of top performers, most of whom were legends destined for the Hall of Fame—Magic Johnson, Michael Jordan, Larry Bird, Charles Barkley, David Robinson, and others. The team dominated the Olympics and captured the fascination of many Americans, particularly young people, and most particularly—Angela. She was now into the NBA. She asked me to take her to watch the Minnesota Timberwolves. I was elated. We were off to the games!

That fall my beautiful eleven-year-old and I went to downtown Minneapolis early on game nights and negotiated with ticket scalpers outside the Target Center. Angela's eyes sparkled as we carried on these slightly nefarious conversations—unless the night was cold. On those frosty evenings, we usually overpaid, buying the first decent seats available.

The Timberwolves rarely won any of the games Angela and I attended the first year. That didn't matter much. The more important thing was that my daughter had a developing understanding and love of the game. In addition, she was enthralled by the Timberwolves Performance Team and carefully observed the cheerleaders' choreographed dance moves. Angela's expanding interest in basketball carried over to other NBA teams and, for a reason I did not question, her favorite team was the San Antonio Spurs. I suspected she was attracted to the color pink in their logo, but she never confirmed my suspicion. Angela did say she thought number 32, Sean Elliott, was "cute."

Throughout the following season we attended a dozen games, using the services of scalpers. The highlight of the second year was a fan event at the Target Center, where Angela met members of the Performance Team. The young women on the team liked Angela, and two of them, in particular, came over to talk with her on breaks during subsequent games. Angela thought their colorful performances were the "best" and their sparkly, fitted costumes were even better. Even though she didn't attend most of the games with us, Linda also enjoyed Angela's enthusiasm and supported her desire to acquire duplicate costumes so she could feel authentic performing the squad cheers at home.

I was skeptical at first about the idea of recreating such skimpy outfits for a twelve-year-old. But Angela and Linda were on a mission, which usually meant I was merely along for the ride. Eventually I shared their excitement, once I was assured that the costume versions for Angela would be more conservative.

Linda spoke to team members who had "adopted" Angela. From them Linda found out the name of the seamstress who created the performance team outfits. When Linda told her about Angela's love for the cheerleaders and their costumes, the seamstress agreed to adapt four of the costumes for Angela. The day we picked them up, she was so excited. I was glad I had gone along with their plan. The joy on Angela's face, seeing the custom-made outfits, and then trying them on, was worth the cost. Now she was one of the "girls." She felt like a real cheerleader and she practiced the cheers for hours in our downstairs family room. The movements were more like dances than cheers, and the vigorous exercise was a huge benefit for anyone with CF.

W HEN WE LEARNED that the 1994/1995 NBA All Star Game was to be held in Minneapolis, Angela and I wanted to be there for the big night in February. Knowing tickets were at a premium and hard to come by unless you were a season ticket holder, we went to the Target Center to buy season tickets. The first level was already sold out, but we left our request to be called if any first-level tickets became available. Angela was anxious to buy the tickets offered, but I told her, "We'll be patient. Don't worry; they'll call us. They won't pass up willing customers for season tickets."

The Wolves had good crowds for a poor team but the games didn't usually sell out. Sure enough, one week later we received the call. We were now season ticket holders, attending the All-Star game. In hindsight, the actual All-Star game was not so special in the scope of things but, now that Angela and I were season ticket holders, we shared so many more father-daughter nights together.

That spring Angela suggested we go to San Antonio to see the Spurs for our Easter vacation. Linda and I had never been there but we'd heard San Antonio was a great vacation spot. We agreed to Angela's adventure. Our trip included two Spurs games, shopping at the Spurs official merchandise store, and a visit to the brand new SeaWorld San Antonio. On the flight to San Antonio, Northwest Airlines mislabeled the tags on Angela's bronchial drainage therapy machine. Her equipment was mistakenly sent to San Diego. We were told the airlines would take a day to deliver the machine to us in San Antonio.

The large air compression machine that powered the therapy vest was two feet high, inside a three-by-three feet metal casing on wheels, with hook-ups for the air hoses. The knobs and dials on the machine had to be adjusted to achieve the right combination of vibration, speed, and force of air into the vest during therapy. The unavailability of the treatment machine for a full day represented a particular freedom we'd not felt before. We were still able to do aerosol treatments, and we could have reverted back to manual bronchial drainage treatments (pounding), if necessary. But we decided, instead, not to do bronchial drainage for one entire day.

Dr. Warwick, and others at the CF Center, had told us that many CF patients were not diligent about carrying out their minimum two therapies per day, but that was not true of Angela. She had not missed a single therapy until our trip to San Antonio. For fourteen years, every single day, she had a minimum of two thirty-minute treatments. When a cold attacked, or she was having a bad day—three, four, five, or more therapies were required to keep her lungs clear. The rigid routine had started with Linda and me, but Angela had quite naturally adopted the discipline. She understood, even if she felt well, the importance of doing therapies on schedule to stay well. Doing so was preventive. Doing so was our ritual. We believed such discipline had kept Angela relatively healthy since the difficult weeks before her CF diagnosis at three months old. We assumed our diligence was one of the reasons she had not been hospitalized since those early days. Her experience was unusual, even remarkable, compared to most CF patients, whose childhoods were intermittently or regularly punctuated by hospitalizations.

Our small family felt carefree in San Antonio, missing therapies for that whole day. We felt somewhat separated from

CF for a brief moment. We were lighthearted "risk takers." Yet I was thankful the following day when the airlines delivered the machine to our hotel, and we were able to return to the regimen that provided the only sense of security we had in our fight against CF.

EDEN PRAIRIE HIGH SCHOOL was one of the largest suburban high schools in Minnesota with more than 2,800 students in four grades. With the school's campus-like setting, outstanding scholastic credentials, and state championship athletic programs, Linda and I wanted to be sure that Angela was not overwhelmed by the size and competitive nature of the school. We talked to her about the number of students in the high school and offered her the option of a smaller, private school. But she wanted to stay with her friends.

Angela was a little shy when she entered ninth grade, but she also exhibited a subtle confidence, poise, and a competitive spirit of her own. As with her therapy regimen, she had a quiet discipline, which she applied effectively in school. She quickly made solid friendships with both boys and girls. Her closest circle of girlfriends numbered about a dozen, but she was virtually inseparable from three girlfriends throughout high school. Angela, Andrea, Marcia, and Lynn did everything together. They giggled about boys and later went on double or triple dates together. They spent entire evenings sitting in a booth at Applebee's or at school events, then talked on the phone or chatted online for hours after they went home.

Linda and I began to notice that Angela's friends called her "Angie," and she now referred to herself as "Angie" with her friends. When we asked her if she preferred to be called Angie, she said that "between us" what we called her didn't matter; she said she liked the name Angela. She might have thought "Angie" sounded more "hip" for high school. Linda continued to call her Angela, and I used both Angie and Angela.

ANGELA HAD NO FORMAL TRAINING in gymnastics and only a little dance experience. But she was determined to join the thirty-member cheerleading squad. In a school the size of Eden Prairie High School, dozens of girls tried out for each available spot on the squad. The school had thousands of fans at major sporting events, so becoming a cheerleader was a prized position and a challenge. Angela quietly began training and practicing in our basement and signed up for a two-day cheerleading camp. More strenuous exercise was a valuable supplement to her daily therapies.

Parents were not allowed to attend the formal cheerleading tryouts. After witnessing the intensity of some parents at high school sporting events, that decision by school officials was probably wise. The night of tryouts, Linda and I dropped off Angie at school and picked her up several hours later. She gave us no indication of how she thought her tryout went. We didn't press her. I presumed she did not want to get our expectations too high before knowing whether she made the cut. Angela knew that making the team meant real work was ahead. Her goal in every endeavor was to put forth her best effort.

The next day Angela, Linda, and I drove to the school together to see the posted results. Linda and I were so excited to see Angela's name on the list. We slapped hands in a high-five and clapped. Angela was less demonstrative, saying, "It's no big deal," but Linda and I knew better. Our daughter allowed her excitement to show through for a moment when our eyes met and we exchanged nods. That was a happy day.

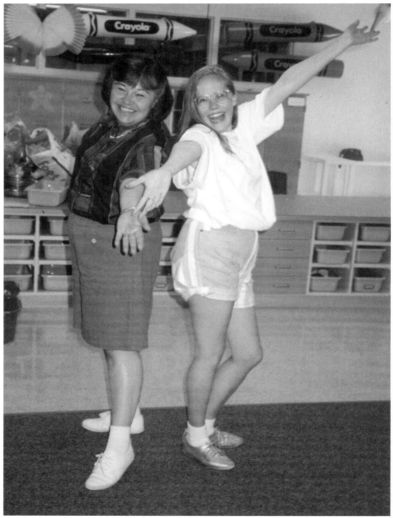

Practicing cheers

Homecoming

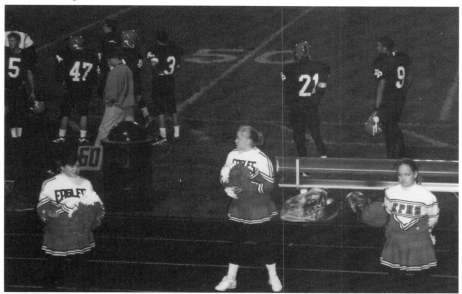

Pam Olson (Mrs. O) says . . .

When Angela Warner walked through my kindergarten classroom door in the fall of 1986, we began a lifelong friendship. In
the coming years, Linda, Angela, and I celebrated birthdays,
Christmases, and the end of each school year together. Our relationship expanded as Angela and I discovered we had several
mutual interests. I'd collected dolls for many years and so had
she. (Angela was fourteen when she surprised me on my fiftieth
birthday with a gift of the American Girl doll, Samantha.)
Angela was a cheerleader, as I had been in high school. I went
to many Eden Prairie High School games to watch her. She was
a spectacular varsity cheerleader. I was so proud of her.

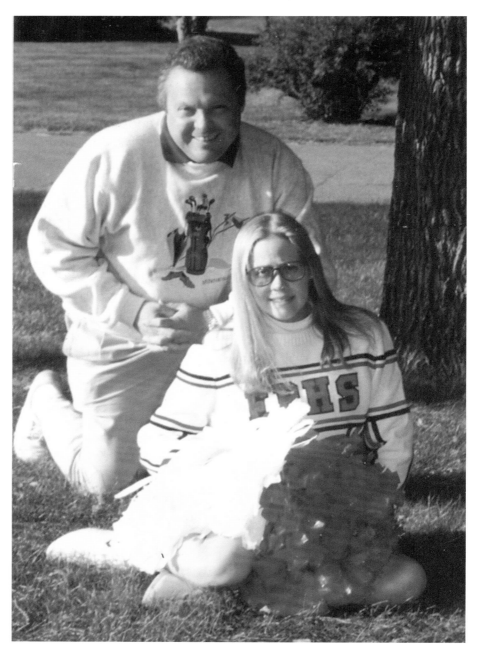

Angie met her first boyfriend, Chris, through an Internet chat line. He was a junior in a high school in Duluth, Minnesota, three hours north of the Twin Cities. Angie assured Linda and me that Chris was a wonderful guy and a handsome football player. A "long distance" romance for a fifteen-year-old seemed just about perfect from my perspective. But Angie had her own plans and she was usually pretty persuasive. Linda and Angela attended a football game Chris's team played in the Twin Cities. Chris passed the test for both mother and daughter. Now he needed the "dad" test.

Angie pushed for a weekend "winter vacation" in Duluth, and, of course, we went. We had absolutely no problem finding a hotel room in March in Duluth. The city is only eighty miles from the nation's undisputed record-breaking cold spot, International Falls. The first night we arrived we had a very pleasant dinner with Chris and his parents. Angie and Chris went to the hotel coffee shop after dinner to get to know each other, and the next afternoon they explored Duluth together. They were a cute couple and it was obvious to me they enjoyed each other's company. But our visit was cut short by an impending major snowstorm. We left Saturday evening instead of Sunday morning, much to Angela's chagrin. We were no more than an hour out of Duluth when the snow began. We had a long drive home in heavy snow with limited visibility.

Angie and Chris only dated a short time—the long-distance aspect of the romance proved limiting—but they remained lifelong friends.

Aₙɢɪᴇ ᴀɴᴅ I ꜱʜᴏᴘᴘᴇᴅ together for her first car shortly after her sixteenth birthday. We visited several used car lots and finally found a three-year-old silver Honda Prelude. The Prelude was a good choice for fun and reliability as she learned to drive. I could see by Angie's face that she loved the car. After a test drive, I told her privately that, no matter what happened, she was not to speak as we negotiated with the salesman in his office.

I had a fair price in mind, but the salesman had other ideas. He used every sales trick to convince me to accept his price. I finally turned to Angela and told her we had to leave. She gave me a shocked look but she complied in smoldering silence. As she was about to work herself into a full bluster halfway to our car, I whispered, "Wait. This ain't over yet."

At that moment the salesman came running across the lot to say our price was acceptable. I refused to return to his office until he agreed to throw a car cover and a service contract into the deal. Angie remained wide-eyed and delighted as we closed the sale. I think Angie and I had even more fun reliving the purchase process than she did driving that car.

I admit, Angela usually won her negotiations with me. We had negotiated many times and many things since she first learned to talk. That day, Angie was impressed to learn a different method of negotiation. She had a newfound respect for patience and the effectiveness of behaving as though the outcome didn't matter. No doubt she'd use that technique with me.

Aɴɢᴇʟᴀ ᴡᴀꜱ ʙᴇᴄᴏᴍɪɴɢ a beautiful young woman. Her glasses were traded for contact lenses and her smile was large and brilliant. She had a charisma that lit up a room. She was blessed with clear, porcelain-smooth skin, just like my mother's. She rarely wore much makeup. Despite her ability to turn heads, Angie did not dress or behave in an attention-seeking manner. Her beauty was natural and her personal style was clean-cut and collegial, low profile and innocent.

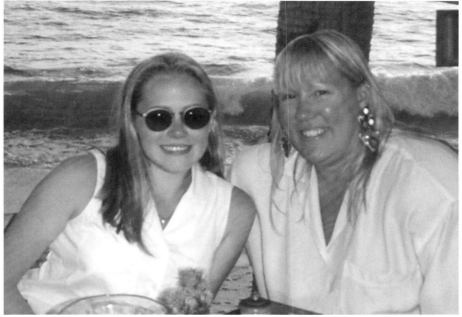

Laguna Beach

Her next boyfriend came along when Angie was a sophomore. As a father, seeing my daughter start to date regularly was not an easy thing, but the day had come. Dan Johnson was a year older than Angie, but Linda and I were comfortable with them being together, especially because Dan put real effort into being respectful to Angie and to us.

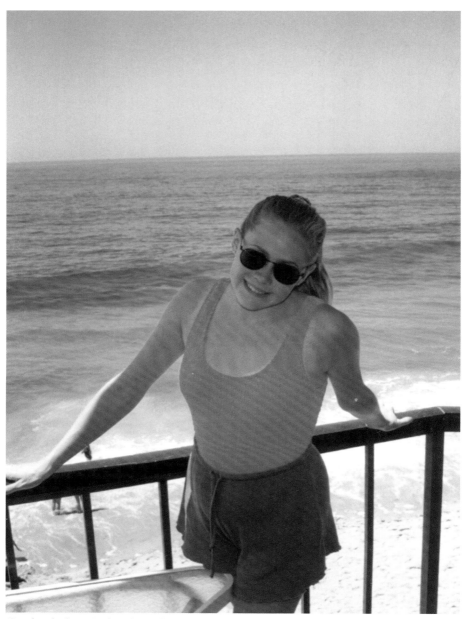

On the deck at Surf and Sand

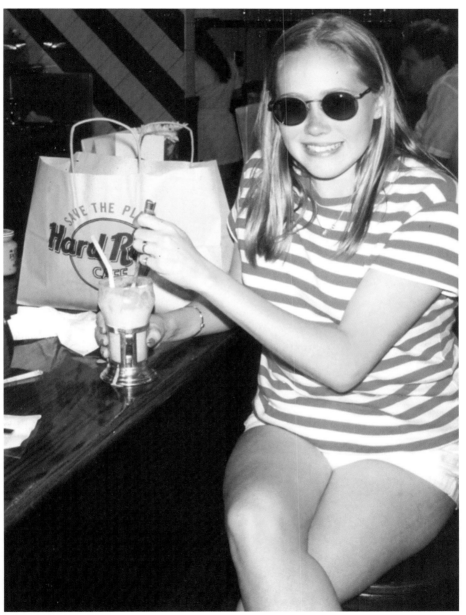

Beverly Hills

After Angie and Dan stopped dating, she met a dashing young man in a jewelry store. He had slick good looks and a confident swagger. Linda and I each sensed he was insincere. I felt quite strongly about the subject, so much so that after their second date I told Angie, "Be careful with this one." She only nodded. I suspected she had already perceived as much on her own, because she didn't go out with him again.

Dan and Angie had stayed good friends, and he introduced her to his friend, J.D. Eisenberg, during Angie's junior year. Angie and J.D. quickly became a busy twosome, going to movies, concerts, fairs, sporting events, and shows. Angie was not the most prompt date, partly due to her need to fit in therapies before going out. But J.D. always waited patiently for her. He was a respectful (a quality I always appreciated) and responsible escort, and they sure seemed to have good times together.

They had been dating for some months when J.D. asked Angie to the senior prom. Linda and I had little idea about the significance of a prom. We both came from small towns with nothing comparable to the Eden Prairie High School prom. At first we did not comprehend the scope of the event, with its formal wear, limousines, promenade marches, all-night chaperoned parties, and an air of blossoming romance. Once we grasped the concept, we wanted Angela to have the most special prom possible.

As a parent of a child with a chronic disease that would mostly likely take her life, I found that dealing with the potential extravagance of a prom night was part of my long-term balancing act. Part of the balance was dealing with immediate short-term pleasure and joy while, at the same time, hoping and planning for the long term. I wanted to instill certain values in my daughter that would serve her throughout her life—things like moderation, earning her own spending money, and living on a budget. I wanted her to understand that, despite our relative prosperity, life had limits, and deferred gratification was often a virtue.

But the other side of the equation was the knowledge that Angela fought a deadly disease every day. She fought hard and never complained. Although this was not discussed in any direct way, by her teenage years, Angie, too, was aware that cystic fibrosis might very well shorten her life. Linda and I wanted our daughter to have the maximum of life experiences we were able to provide. When the time came for proms, vacations, having a car, and other experiences, we chose the latter course most often, and we were grateful that we could. We never regretted doing so.

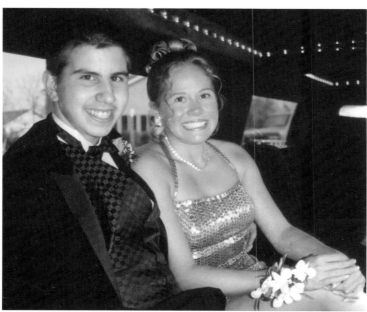

Prom night with Angie and J.D.

J.D. Eisenberg says . . .

Angie was extra special. She was my first girlfriend, and she had the most beautiful smile I'd ever seen. She had this amazing glow about her. On our first date we saw the movie, *The Little Mermaid.* On Valentine's Day, Angie made a poster with glow-in-the-dark stars that spelled out "I love you." She snuck into my house and hung the poster on the ceiling above where I slept, so I'd see it when I went to bed.

I couldn't believe she was actually my girlfriend. She was way out of my league, but that didn't matter to her. We enjoyed movies, concerts, mini golf, and her favorite: dancing. As much as I hated dancing, Angie always made those high school dances fun. She kept tickets and other little things from everything we did and put them in a scrapbook. I didn't understand why creating a memory book was such a big deal to her back then.

Even when we were not dating, we remained great friends. She often brought me to family events. My love for Angie went beyond being my girlfriend and a best friend. She cared about everyone. I'd do anything for her, and I knew she'd have done anything for me.

The night of Angie's first prom was magical. She was beautiful in a blue, sequined dress. Her hair was swept up and her smile was radiant. Five couples met at J.D.'s parents' home to be whisked off in a super-stretch limousine. The parents were all present to watch the couples drive away. At the prom, parents came to watch the Grand March, as each couple was introduced to the cheering crowd. After the prom, Angela joined her friends back at J.D.'s home for a party.

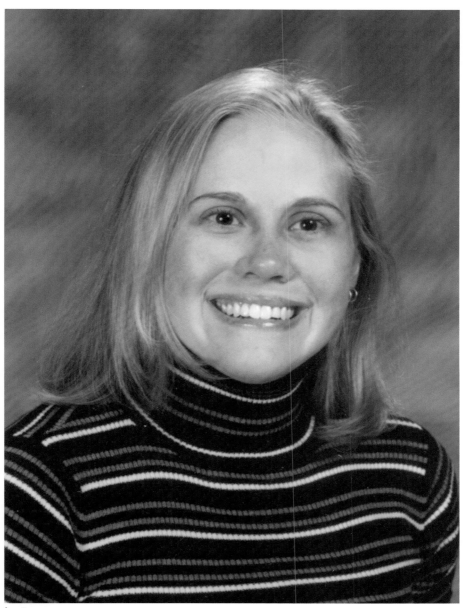

Junior year

OVERALL, Angie's entire junior year in high school was blessed. Her health was stable; she was a popular and bright student; she had a great boyfriend, adoring parents, and she was a cheerleader. Life was good. Her time was filled with school events, sporting events, movies, concerts, parties, and dinners at Applebee's with J.D. When J.D.'s graduation approached, she created a "memory book" as a present for him, filling a scrapbook with pictures and other reminders of their year together. She had saved theatre and concert ticket stubs, and much more, and she included a written narrative to go with the memories. Although Angie and J.D. stopped dating soon after his graduation, they continued an enduring and tender friendship.

As ANGIE BEGAN HER SENIOR YEAR, a new boyfriend entered her life. Craig was a year younger than Angie, and Linda and I teased her about dating a "younger man." But Craig was mature beyond his years with a stated goal of becoming valedictorian of his class, which meant achieving nothing less than an A in every class from seventh grade until the end of high school. He was also handsome and a star diver on the swim team.

Craig and Angie dated through Angie's final year of high school. Craig was yet another outstanding young man with whom Angela remained close friends even after they stopped dating.

During the football season, Angela was having trouble with sinus allergies. She was now seeing a different doctor at the CF Center. Her new physician, Dr. Eddy, was a colleague of Dr. Warwick. He wanted to put Angela in the hospital to perform a procedure that would clear her sinuses, especially a compacted area under her right eye. This was a procedure that could have been done on an outpatient basis for a person who did not have cystic fibrosis.

Angela "toughed it out" until after the football season, then went into the hospital in November for three days during the Thanksgiving weekend, without telling Craig or any of her friends. She had to arrive at the hospital the day before the procedure to be started on IV antibiotics. All her CF therapies continued while she was an inpatient. The procedure was successful, and Angie was back in school the following Monday. However, at a follow-up clinic appointment, we learned that pseudomonas had shown up in her lab results for the first time.

I had dreaded the day we might hear that Angie had pseudomonas. I learned about this "marker" from the doctors, my own research, and books I'd read, such as Frank Deford's book, *Alex: The Life of A Child*. The majority of people with cystic fibrosis are eventually chronically infected with pseudomonas.

Pseudomonas aeruginosa bacterium doesn't typically infect healthy tissue, but the bacteria will infect any compromised tissue, such as the lungs of those with cystic fibrosis. And once present, pseudomonas is there to stay, never to be eradicated, only controlled, hopefully. Linda and I held onto the wish that Angela was the exception to that dire prediction—the one in a thousand, or whatever huge number was quoted, whose pseudomonas went away. However, even when attacked with aggressive antibiotics, pseudomonas is able to survive in remote areas of the lungs and even hide in other tissues to return later to the airways.

I was grateful that Angela had lived to age seventeen without contracting pseudomonas. Now I was worried about the implications of the bacteria's arrival in Angela's body. Monitoring the level and type of pseudomonas became a major focus of each future quarterly clinic visit.

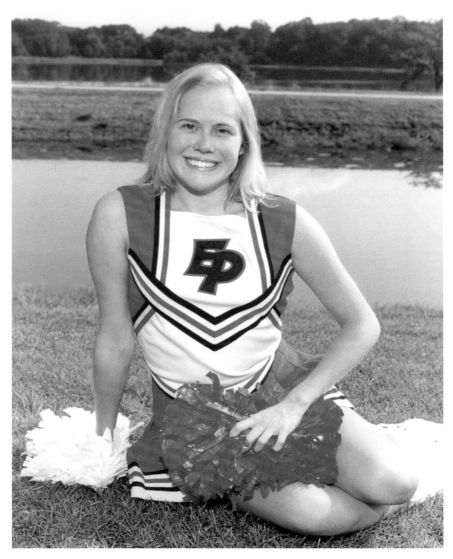

DURING HER HIGH SCHOOL YEARS, Angie was able to excel academically, enjoy school activities, cheerleading, sporting events, and social aspects. She did all these activities without sharing with others that she lived day-to-day with cystic fibrosis and the exhausting multiple-therapy regimen that took hours of each day.

Sometimes, when she was fighting a cold or infection, she had a cough for weeks at a time that sounded like her lungs were being coughed up. For years, Linda and I heard these horrible coughs, or listened for them, holding our fear that they might turn into a far more serious problem.

Angela lived as though she was not aware of a truth that, unless a cure was found, the future meant things were going to become worse for her. The courage and strength of children and young adults with CF is inspiring. I know there were times when Angela was worn out or depressed by everything CF entailed, but Linda and I saw this disquieting look only occasionally in our daughter's eyes, and it was never visible to the rest of the world.

Angela emerged from high school as a competent, mature and beautiful young woman. By graduation night I was sorry, as I know she was a little, too, that high school was ending. Because of the size of the 1999 senior class, the graduation ceremony was held in Northrop Auditorium on the main campus of the University of Minnesota. I had attended many classes and events at Northrop, including my college graduation from the Carlson School of Management, so I felt a little nostalgic to be back there for Angie's ceremony.

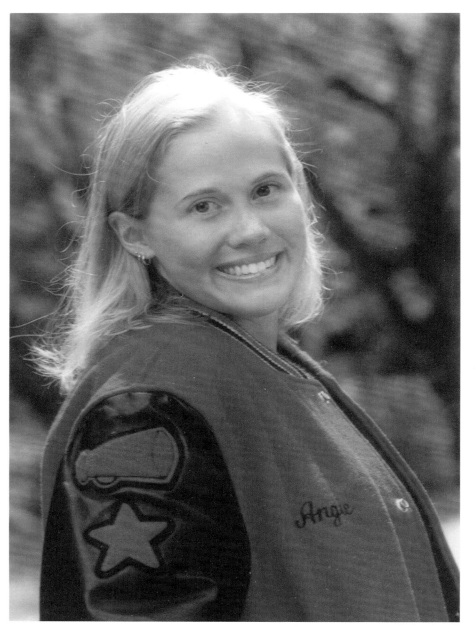

Photograph courtesy Steve Lucas Photography

Linda and I, along with Craig, Linda's mother, and several thousand others in attendance, watched as our little girl received her diploma and graduated with honors. A reception followed outside the auditorium. I looked up just as Angela emerged from the crowd of graduates and saw us waiting to greet and congratulate her. She came running and jumped into my arms. I swung her around with joy and hugged her as tight as I could without hurting her.

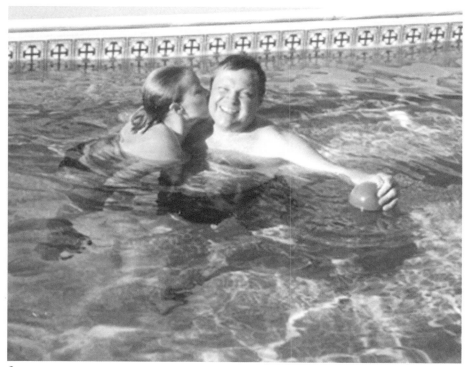

Summer 1999

EXPLORING
OPTIONS

ngela decided to attend Normandale Community College in the nearby city of Bloomington, Minnesota. The college was twenty minutes from our home, so she could easily commute. Her goal was to complete some basic classes there without a disruption in her health care, social life, and family. Linda and I encouraged Angie to explore her options and discover her true interests. With our many trips to the ocean and SeaWorld, we were not surprised when she expressed interest in becoming a marine biologist.

I appreciated her enthusiasm and fascination with marine life, but I suspected her interest might diminish when she discovered the true nature of what biologists often do with some of the creatures they study. Linda and I supported Angie's passions and discussed the possibility with her of spending her final two years of college in California. Many schools there had marine biology programs and a desirable location near the ocean.

We had gone to Laguna Beach at least once every year since Angela was five years old. Her love for the ocean was evident and continued to grow from her first visit as she ran along the beach and swam. In her teenage years, she sat for long periods, watching the waves from the deck or while sunning on the beach. We usually made an event of being well positioned on our deck or at a restaurant for the best view of the setting sun and the feel of the ocean breeze.

Angie and I continued to share our walks on the beach after dark. At times I might have preferred to relax after running around all day but my energetic teenage daughter was always ready for our beach walks. How could I resist? Stars were always abundant as Angela and I walked arm in arm, talking about the universe. Distant lights from the hotels shone on the beach, yet the night was dark, almost eerie. We marveled at how the ocean waves had been washing ashore endlessly for millions of years. They changed over time, but they never stopped. She stared in silence and hugged my arm as the white-foam waves rolled toward us.

THE SUMMER OF 1999, Angela, Craig and their friends were busy enjoying their last summer together before starting college. In spite of Angie's busy social schedule, she and Linda still spent regular time with each other every day. They were truly best friends. On weekdays they prepared lunch together so they were settled in their chairs, ready to watch *All My Children*, make fun of the story line, and evaluate the men on the show. In addition to the daily lunch/soap opera ritual, they frequently went "malling" together. The first enclosed shopping mall in the world was built in nearby Edina in 1956 and, by now, the Twin Cities area was the home of many more malls, including the super-mall, the Mall of America, which attracted people from around the world. Angie and Linda were world-class shoppers who took advantage of the close proximity to the megamall.

Once or twice a week, Angie joined Linda and me for family dinners at restaurants or we'd grill at home. She loved my thick, barbequed hamburgers. (Angela always had good taste.) And, with Dad, she also had expensive taste. Her restaurant of choice with dates was a neighborhood place like Applebee's, but on family dinner night, she opted for a restaurant with great steaks, shrimp, lobster, or grilled swordfish. A rich dessert was always shared. Taking Angela and Linda to fine restaurants on a regular basis seemed like mini-vacations to me.

Angela took a couple of road trips with friends that summer. One was to Madison, to visit friends at the University of Wisconsin. By then, the compressor unit for the vest she used for therapy was smaller than the original version and could be lifted by a handle like a large suitcase. Angie preferred to rent a room by herself and have the bellman help her load and unload the equipment. She was able to maintain her privacy and carry out her therapies as needed.

We took our annual, highlight-of-the-summer, ten-day trip to Laguna Beach that year in August, returning to the Surf and Sand Hotel. An added advantage for me was getting away from the ragweed season in Minnesota for a short time. The trip also signaled the end of the summer. Angela started at Normandale within a week of our return.

A new school year always meant a new schedule with added intensity to make sure her required CF therapies and medications fit into the school day. Angela now carried out the many responsibilities of her therapies, but Linda and I tried to support her by helping in any way we could to make the cumbersome routine easier. Linda prepared Angie's daily medications and continued to clean the therapy equipment.

The first semester at Normandale went smoothly. Angela usually stayed at school to study. Linda and I rarely saw her do homework but her grades were always A's or B's.

ANGELA WAS FEELING PRETTY GOOD until February of 2000 when a bad cold turned into pneumonia. Dr. Eddy advised her to check into the hospital for a "tune-up." We were aware that "routine" tune-ups were not unusual for someone with CF who contracted occasional pulmonary infections or other symptoms. We had also been told to expect Angie to lose at least two to three percent of her lung function per year in adulthood. Linda and I looked at Angela's first tune-up as a potential opportunity to give her lungs an extra degree or two of function that might have been lost as she became older. Angie had remained diligent about therapies and clinic visits (especially with the concern about pseudomonas), but tune-ups were inevitable.

Angela did not want Craig or any of her friends to know about her hospitalization, so Linda and I were her only visitors during her weeklong stay. Linda spent a couple of nights with Angela until she felt more comfortable. She received IV antibiotics, inhaled medications from a nebulizer, took her normal dietary enzymes and supplements, and had added sessions of her regular therapies. When she was able, Angela read, watched television or chatted online with her friends. She quickly felt healthy again and only missed a few classes.

After one week, Angela was allowed to go home as long as she was willing to continue to receive IV antibiotics for a couple of weeks through a PICC line placed under her arm. The antibiotics had to be injected with a syringe four to six times a day. Angela did not like this part.

A PICC line is a peripherally inserted central catheter made of soft plastic. This can be used over a prolonged period, usually no more than thirty days, to administer intravenous medication. A PICC line is especially useful for the delivery of powerful antibiotics to fight infections like pseudomonas. The line is inserted into a large vein where strong medicine is less irritating. The line was held in place with sutures and the insertion site was covered with a clear sterile dressing. After Angela's discharge from the hospital, she had to be careful when showering to keep the site dry. She disliked the PICC-line tubing hanging under her arm, but she was happy to be out of the hospital.

Linda and I were trained to do the IV injections. The process involved several steps. To help keep the PICC line open and free of blood clots, we had to flush saline solution into the line before each injection. The antibiotics were followed with a small amount of heparin, an anticoagulant. The heparin lock kept the IV unclogged between infusions. We were warned to watch for redness, swelling, leakage or other complications. Angela paid close attention to the training and watched closely to make sure Linda and I did each step correctly.

Angie went back to school and was enjoying her social life. She felt particularly good after the PICC line was removed. She and Craig broke up sometime around her birthday in March, leaving Angie more time to spend with her friends, Andrea, Lynn, and J.D. She dated a couple of young men briefly after Craig, including a well-mannered, handsome high school friend named Steve, but none were "the" relationship.

DURING THE SUMMER OF 2000, St. Paul, Minnesota, was celebrating hometown boy and cartoonist Charles Shultz who had died earlier that year. Bronze sculptures of eleven Peanuts characters adorned the St. Paul riverfront and seventy-five large colorful statues of Snoopy were placed in various spots throughout the city. Linda's sister Mary, who lived in Denver, was a huge fan and collector of Snoopy memorabilia. Linda and Angie decided to do something special for Mary since she was about to turn fifty. They decided to take pictures of every Snoopy in the exhibit. Angie asked J.D. to be their chauffeur for their photo shoot. He was an enthusiastic assistant. Together they mapped out the locations of the statues and, over several afternoons, took photos of every Snoopy. Angie put the pictures in a book for Mary, writing captions for each one. Mary was ecstatic!

Marcia Gallant says . . .

After completing my freshman year of college at the University of Oklahoma I had a plane ticket to visit my friends in Minnesota for a week in the summer of 2000. The person I wanted to stay with most was Angie. When I asked if I could stay a week with her, she hesitated but agreed. I didn't know what the hesitation was about, but I did recall I had never before spent a night at her house. Sure, our group of friends hung out over at Angie's plenty of times, but not overnight. Not thinking more about it, I continued planning my visit.

Angie called back a week later, and told me there was something I needed to know before staying at her house. She told me she had cystic fibrosis—and breathing treatments to do every day, sometimes for more than an hour. The true shocker to me was that she swore me to secrecy. Most of our friends had known each other since elementary school, yet I had come into the group only three years earlier. How could I possibly be the first to know about this? I recalled the sleepovers we had in high school; I could not fathom how none of us knew Angie had to do breathing treatments before she came over for the night. She was a cheerleader... how was that possible with CF? Grateful that she allowed me in on this secret in her life, I agreed not to tell anyone.

During that weeklong visit, I didn't actually think much about Angie's disease. She disappeared into another room for an hour or so, and I passed the time chatting with friends online. I tried to give Angie as much time and space as she needed for her treatments. The week passed too quickly, and I went home to Oklahoma. I kept Angie's secret.

DURING ANGIE'S SECOND YEAR at Normandale, she began to focus on a different career choice—interior design—which I thought was much more consistent with Angie's personality than marine biology. Linda and I always trusted Angie's opinions on color coordination or decorating options. Even as a little girl, she always had great instincts. Angie focused on her new academic direction with passion. She took the available classes at Normandale and also enrolled in an independent correspondence course in interior design.

During that winter, Angie began using her entrepreneurial skills on the Internet. She had long been a collector of dolls. She began with the original Care Bears during the 1980s and extended her interest to the American Girl dolls during the late 1990s. She had seven American Girl dolls and many accessories. Angie started selling different items on eBay but quickly saw that the "real action" was in American Girl dolls and animated Disney movies. She discovered that a lot of the American Girl doll accessories, and some of the dolls, sold on the Internet for more than the retail cost and, at a minimum, more than the discounted prices often found. So, with a little financing from Dad, Angela entered the online business world. She purchased accessories randomly on the Internet and did enough research to know if an item was underpriced. She began to build a small inventory. She attended American Girl doll shows in the area to buy dolls and accessories at reduced prices. She listed and sold her products on eBay, making certain she saved enough of the sales proceeds to replenish her inventory.

Angela wasn't feeling well in February 2001 and was admitted to the hospital for another tune-up. Angie hated more than feared another hospitalization. As usual, she didn't want anyone to know she was there. Being in the hospital was boring; nurses and other clinicians interrupted her all the time for all kinds of things, her computer worked slowly on the hospital's dial-up connection—so keeping track of her online business was harder and, of course, she disliked everything about having a PICC line again.

Her one pleasure as an inpatient was the large caramel roll that Linda or I picked up each morning from the hospital cafeteria. Angie endured the inpatient process and soon went back to school, wearing clothing that covered any evidence of the PICC line that had to stay under her arm for the next couple of weeks while we carried out the required antibiotic injections.

As Angie neared completion of her second year of college, she continued working on her correspondence course. She had taken all of the courses she could at Normandale. The time had come for her to look to the next stage of her education. She still liked the idea of attending college on the West Coast. She did her homework, researching several colleges in Southern California. She decided on the interior design program at Mesa College in San Diego. Her plan was to go to Mesa for one year, then apply for a transfer to the University of California at San Diego (UCSD) to complete her bachelor's degree. UCSD was a great school located on a hill in La Jolla, overlooking the Pacific Ocean. Because non-residents of California were unlikely to gain entrance into UCSD, the advantage of a year at Mesa was to establish Angie's residency in California.

After long and thoughtful discussions, we agreed on a plan. We would find a three-bedroom apartment in La Jolla. Linda would relocate with Angela, stay with her for most of every month, and I'd come out for at least ten days each month. Linda and Angie would then return to Minnesota during school breaks. Linda and I had occasionally spoken about the possibility of retiring one day to Laguna Beach or La Jolla, so we viewed this as an opportunity to see if La Jolla suited us. This was a big move that would put a lot of pressure on all of us, but Linda and I thought the plan was a sensible way to fulfill Angie's dreams and do some experimentation for ourselves.

Angie would continue her regular medical care at the University of Minnesota CF Center, returning to Minnesota quarterly for her check-ups. We arranged to use the Cystic Fibrosis Center at UCSD for any emergency care. Angie's doctor at the University of Minnesota CF Center affirmed that the UCSD CF Center's reputation was quite good.

We began our search for an apartment during a trip to Laguna Beach in May 2001. After looking at several options, we found a beautiful place with a panoramic view of Mt. Soledad. The apartment was a ten-minute drive to the village of La Jolla and ten minutes to Mesa College. Angie and Linda planned to move there in August in time for the start of school.

EVEN AS THE MOVE PLANS PROGRESSED, Angie developed a closer friendship with another young man. Josh Rasmusson had been a familiar face at our door since Angie was in high school. He delivered pizza for Domino's, and our household was a regular customer. Josh later confessed that he always wanted to deliver to the Warner house, just in case Angie answered the door. Their friendship had been evolving for more than a year but had been especially close since the early spring. They got together every couple of weeks for movies or meals, often with Linda, since she and Angie were so much like girlfriends.

One evening in late May, the three of them were lingering over a meal at Old Chicago when Linda asked Josh and Angie why they didn't date. Josh and Angie both laughed. He said, "That would be like dating my sister!"

But the idea must have taken root because by July 2001, they were together every day. When they weren't in each other's company, Angie and Josh sent each other emails or online instant messages. He sent her flowers, and she encouraged him to move to California too, so they could still be together.

Once again, Angela had chosen a great young man who was polite, a hard-worker and obviously well-parented. Linda and I enjoyed Josh's company so much that the four of us did things together as well. We invited him to join us on future family vacations.

ANGELA BECAME MORE EXCITED about her upcoming move to the West Coast once Josh decided to relocate there as well. To earn extra money to finance his move, Josh decided to try dealing in American Girl dolls and Disney DVDs, too. He was impressed with Angie's successful part-time eBay business. She

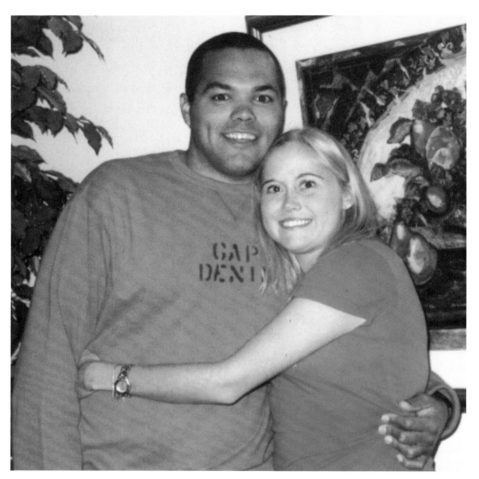

Josh and Angie

helped him with his purchases and sales and had goodhearted fun with him in their shared business rivalry. With careful planning and money savings, his plan was to be on the West Coast by October or November. Angie joked that she'd have to give up pizza for a while in California because she couldn't bear to have anyone but Josh deliver it to her door.

Josh adopted a pug he named Beyonce. Angie helped Josh with his dog, and she wanted a puppy, too; she had already chosen a preferred breed and name. She wanted a female Maltese, and she planned to name her puppy Torrance, after the lead character, a cheerleader, in the movie *Bring It On*.

I reminded her about my allergy to dogs. She asked, "Can I get one if the dog lives at Josh's apartment?"

I couldn't say no to that. Angie did the research, but locating a female Maltese turned out to be a challenge. She began an extensive online search.

The rest of the summer was busy planning the move, arranging to transport Angie's car and Linda's car to California as well as purchasing the necessary furniture. One by one, the pieces seemed to fall into place.

During the last days before the big move, Angie scheduled special goodbye visits with friends and relatives between packing and spending time with Josh and his puppy. Some days, she ordered pizza delivery from Domino's just to see Josh in the middle of the day. She made time for last-minute shopping and fun at the Mall of America with her twelve-year-old friend, Jackie, and Jackie's sister, Mariana, lunch with Craig, swimming with J.D., a dentist appointment, a pedicure and hair appointment, a concert, and several movies. She packed a lot of activity into a short time.

Jackie Bordes says…

Angie appeared at a time in my life when I really needed someone to rely on. I was six and Angie was sixteen when I met her at J.D.'s graduation. She was so nice to me. I became instantly attached to her. She told me she had always wanted a little sister. After that, she came to our house a lot and played games with me that my sister wouldn't. She's the only person besides my mom whose lap I ever sat on. I considered Angie part of my family. When a friend of mine was playing with us one day, I became upset and began to cry. I was afraid Angie would like my friend more than she liked me. She pulled me onto her lap and told me, "No one can ever take your place." She continued to say sweet, soothing things to me until I was smiling again.

Angie took me to movies I wanted to see, even if she had already seen them. She took me shopping and out to eat at Planet Hollywood. I liked hanging out with her in her room, listening to music. I wished I had as many pairs of shoes as Angie had–her closet had stacks of boxes.

I never once saw her unhappy. She was honestly the nicest person. She accepted people for who they were and didn't judge anyone. I have always wanted to be like Angie.

Jackie Bordes was named the 2007-2008 National American Miss Minnesota Junior Teen. Angie and J.D. sponsored Jackie for her first national pageant when she was seven.

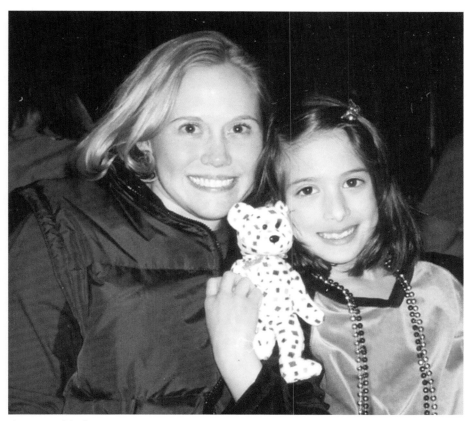

Angie and Jackie

THE
SECRET

As Angie's relationship with Josh took on a deeper commitment, she hinted to him from time to time that she had a secret she would someday share with him. The only clues she gave were that she was "not perfect" and that she was sure he would someday "get sick" of her. She told Josh that knowing her secret would make clear why she had decided she would not marry or have children. She did say that if anyone could change her mind about getting married, he'd be the one, adding, "That is, of course, if after you know my reasons for not wanting to get married, you still want to be with me."

Josh didn't press Angie to say more, but one evening in early August when he was at our house watching a movie, she decided the time had come to tell him her secret. She tried several times to start the conversation, but became more flustered with each attempt. Finally she told Josh that she couldn't tell him face to face. They agreed to talk online as soon as he was home.

So, with the aid of technology, Angie was able to tell Josh her secret. Their extended conversation had several long pauses between messages. (I was, of course, not privy at the time to the exchange below.)

JOSH: So, are you nervous?

ABW: No.

JOSH: Good. Let's hear it out then.

ABW: I don't know.

JOSH: You must tell me.

ABW: Why'd you ask me if Marcia knows?

JOSH: Cuz I figured I could get it out of her. But even if I could, I wouldn't want to hear it from her. I want to hear it from you. It's OK; nothing changes between us by your telling me. Well, the fact that I know changes, but we don't.

JOSH: What is it you want to tell me?

JOSH: Angie...

ABW: Why don't you tell me the worst thing you've thought of is? Cuz then if it's not that bad I would feel better telling you.

JOSH: I'm not going to do that.

ABW: Why not?

JOSH: Because, what if I was right? or if I am completely off base? I would feel like an idiot either way. Nothing. Nothing will change us Angie. You have nothing to worry about.

ABW: But it would be easier if I knew you were expecting something worse.

JOSH: Well, maybe I'm expecting something bad because you are having such a hard time telling me. But something bad to you might not be a big thing for me. I don't want to play guessing games. Please just tell me.

JOSH: I'm starting to worry. I don't like this feeling.

ABW: Well don't worry. OK, if I tell you, you have to promise me something.

JOSH: OK

Angie: You can't tell anyone else. I mean, no one else would probably care, but it's not something I tell a lot of people.

JOSH: It's no one else's business but ours.

ABW: You should feel really special that I am telling you this because the only other person who's ever known outside my family is Marcia, and that's only because she stayed with us last year.

JOSH: I feel special all the time I am with you.

ABW: OK. You know how you said the only thing that could make you break up with me is if I had some kind of mental condition and I could never love you?

JOSH: I remember. And it's true.

ABW: Well, I do have a condition, but it's not mental and it's not going to stop me from loving you because, like I said I think I already do and I meant it.

JOSH: What's your condition?

[Long pause]

ABW: It's called cystic fibrosis. Ever heard of it?

JOSH: Yes. I'm not sure exactly what it is though.

ABW: It's an inherited respiratory disease. Not really inherited, but genetic.

JOSH: How does it affect you?

ABW: It doesn't affect me as much as it does most people who have it.

JOSH: Is it life threatening?

ABW: For example, my dad has a client whose son has CF too and the kid is in the hospital like every freakin' month. I haven't been in the hospital since I was 3 months old, except for when I had surgery two years ago, but that was completely unrelated.

JOSH: How does it affect you in everyday life?

ABW: The reason I had to tell Marcia when she stayed with us, and why I have to tell you so that you can stay with us, I have to do something called therapy two or three times a day.

JOSH: What do you do?

ABW: What CF does is, it blocks some chloride channel and makes the mucus in your lungs thicker, so therapy is this machine that vibrates your lungs to help clear the mucus.

JOSH: Does it hurt?

ABW: No, not at all, and it's actually kind of a good thing to have to do during the school year because Lord knows I would never get all my reading done otherwise, that's when I do most of my homework.

JOSH: I like to study at night.

ABW: Good for you.

JOSH: I'm at this web site.

ABW: OK

JOSH: I hate to type this, but it says that 50% of people with CF live into their 30s.

JOSH: What about you?

ABW: It's higher than that, and I'm a lot healthier than most CF patients are by the time they are 20. My doctor is always impressed because my lungs have no damage.

JOSH: Are you projected to live a normal lifespan?

ABW: Well no, probably not, but a lot closer than most people with CF.

JOSH: There are things I want to ask you.

ABW: So ask.

JOSH: I feel weird typing 'em.

ABW: Just ask. Nothing is weird this late at night, trust me.

JOSH: OK. At least your intelligence isn't affected. That's a good thing.

JOSH: Is your sweat thick and sticky?

ABW: No.

JOSH: Prone to infections?

ABW: More prone to lung infections than most people, yeah, but I think I've only had two or three in my life.

JOSH: Proper growth?

ABW: Well except for being kind of small-chested, yeah :) But I don't think that has anything to do with CF. LOL

JOSH: Small chested…whatever. Nice, they are nice. I'm a guy. I know these things.

ABW: OK :)

JOSH: Digestive problems?

ABW: Nope. I've hardly ever had digestive problems. I used to get stomachaches when I was little, but not anymore.

JOSH: Reproductive problems?

ABW: I wouldn't know that since I've never tried to get pregnant;

I've generally tried to avoid it, ya know. :-P

JOSH: I would hope so.

ABW: Most CF women don't have reproductive problems. That affects men with CF more.

JOSH: It says here that you have a chance for reduced fertility.

ABW: Yeah. Besides, I'm not having kids anyway, that's probably a good thing.

JOSH: This is true.

JOSH: Do you have loose fatty stools?

ABW: That would be a digestive problem, so no.

JOSH: I didn't make that up.

ABW: Yeah, but I already told you I don't have digestive problems.

JOSH: Do you take medication besides the therapy?

ABW: Yeah, just some pills, to lower the risk of infection.

JOSH: Do you do therapy every day?

ABW: Yeah, at least twice a day, sometimes three times.

JOSH: When?

ABW: When I get up and before bed, in the afternoon if I have time, which I usually don't.

JOSH: How long does each one take?

ABW: 30 minutes

JOSH: You never tell anyone about you having CF?

ABW: No. No one needs to know really, except Marcia. I wanted her to be able to stay here.

JOSH: Good thing you don't have the digestive bit—"frequent foul smelling stools."

ABW: LOL. Yeah.

JOSH: Beyonce [his dog] has that one covered.

JOSH: So this is why it takes you a long time to get ready?

ABW: LOL. In the morning, yeah, because it's an extra half hour. Sometimes I do one in the afternoon when I get ready, if I have a cold or my allergies are bugging me, but usually in the afternoon I'm just slow.

JOSH: I don't know if it's just cuz I am [going to be] staying with you, or just because you wanted to tell me, but thank you so much for telling me.

ABW: Both.

FINDING HOME

When the August move-day finally arrived, Angela was excited but somewhat apprehensive, too. The entire relocation was completed smoothly in the middle of the month. We were able to go directly from the airport to the auto transport drop-off, where the cars had just arrived a few hours earlier. The furniture had been delivered the day before our arrival so everything was there when we got to the apartment. Over the next ten days, we unpacked, and Angie and Linda were fairly settled in before I returned to Minnesota. Our first separation, therefore, was only a week or so. My girls flew home for Labor Day weekend.

Josh had not seen Angie for more than two and a half weeks so he came to the airport with me to pick up Angie and Linda.

Angie emerged from the plane with a big smile and a great tan. With her blonde hair blowing in the breeze, she looked like she'd spent her life as a "California girl." She looked so happy. At a clinic appointment the next day at the CF Center, we were pleased to hear Dr. Eddy say that Angela's lungs looked as good as a "normal" person's. The rest of her stay included a couple of trips to the Minnesota State Fair. The short visit went too quickly and, as I hugged my wife and daughter goodbye, I promised to be with them in California on September 13.

The next ten days went well for Angie, despite a cough. She said she liked school for the most part and looked forward to Josh's move to California. She and Linda went apartment shopping for him and found him a place about two miles away. He agreed to come to California in late September to check out the apartment they had found for him. Meanwhile, I spent my time working ahead at my office so I could comfortably be out of the office ten days of the month.

T WO DAYS BEFORE MY FLIGHT to California, Americans woke up to images of airplanes flying into the World Trade Center and the Pentagon. A fourth plane crashed into a field in Pennsylvania. Around the country and the world, everyone was making contact with their distant loved ones on September 11, 2001. We were no different; the phone was my family connection as we remained riveted to the television on opposite sides of the country. I wanted to be with my wife and daughter, but now there was uncertainty about when airports would be functioning again.

The two days until the thirteenth felt like weeks. While I waited in line to check in for my flight on September 13, word spread through the airport that a potential terrorist threat was uncovered at La Guardia Airport in New York. Within minutes, an announcement came that commercial planes were grounded. I wasn't able to fly from the Twin Cities to San Diego until two days later.

UPON MY ARRIVAL IN LA JOLLA, I could see that Angela was not feeling well. Her smile wasn't as ready, and she looked pale. I was not certain whether her less-than-cheerful emotions were the result of a health condition, missing Josh, or the events of 9/11. But the contrast in her state of mind and energy level from only two weeks earlier was evident. She also had a rough cough. Because Linda and I both experienced some congestion and breathing discomfort as well, I suspected at first that the chemicals used to clean the carpeting in the apartment might be the cause. But Angie needed to be seen by a doctor.

Linda and I went to the ER at UCSD with Angela. Once sputum cultures and a chest x-ray were done, she was given oral antibiotics and a follow-up clinic appointment for two days later with the head of their CF Center. We were told that the cultures were clear, showing no pseudomonas. I pointed out to the physician that Angela had tested positive for pseudomonas in quarterly lab tests for years, and we'd always been told pseudomonas didn't go away. But the doctor did not appear concerned about the inconsistency.

In general, the clinicians at the UCSD clinic had a markedly different style of treatment from what we were accustomed to at the University of Minnesota CF Center. The California clinic emphasized lifestyle more than aggressive preventive care for people living with CF. Our family's painstaking adherence to a rigorous therapy discipline that had become Angie's way of life had always provided us with a certain reassurance that we were doing everything we could to protect her health. The more casual approach of the UCSD CF clinic did not provide the same level of relative comfort. We left the clinic feeling slightly uneasy.

During my entire ten-day stay, Angie seemed tense. Linda told me Angie had been busy with her classes and the two of them had spent most of their time getting settled in the apartment, becoming familiar with the neighborhood and looking for an apartment for Josh. Even though Linda was living with her, Angie was lonely. I learned later that she and Josh had a writing journal they sent back and forth, recording their more intimate thoughts. Angela shared with Josh her doubts about her move to California. Although I had sensed Angela was questioning her decision to leave Minnesota, she was not yet ready to tell me how she felt. At one point I advised her that if she was having second thoughts, she shouldn't be encouraging Josh to move to California.

Angie hadn't been back to her classes since 9/11. Her energy and enthusiasm only surfaced when I privately suggested to her that we plan a surprise party for Linda's fiftieth birthday the next month. I suggested we invite Linda's mother, Bernelda, and her godmother, Sister Dorothy. They could fly out with me when I returned in October. Each had only been on an airplane once before, so Linda would not expect them to fly to California. Angie became excited and said Josh could come out then, and the two of them could decorate the apartment. I agreed to be responsible for our guests and the Minnesota end. Angie and I were certain Linda would love our plan. We pledged secrecy to each other. I suspected keeping the party a surprise would be easier for me than Angie. But, she was great; she stuck to our confidential pact.

For the rest of my stay, Angie was in slightly better spirits. I continued to try to figure out what else might be going on with her. And, of course, we continued to watch the television coverage following September eleventh.

On October 2, I was back in Minnesota, talking on the phone with Angie. I heard a trace of apprehension in her voice as she finally asked "would it be all right" if she returned "home" to Minnesota. I could tell she had been agonizing about proposing a return to Minnesota less than two months after moving to California. She was aware of how much work and expense had gone into the move. But the tone in her voice told me this was not the time to question her decision. I immediately said, "Yes, yes," and that I "would love" to bring her back to Minnesota. I heard the relief in her voice.

After more talking over the next few days, we decided together that Angela would stay in California until after Linda's birthday party. Angie would then fly home with Josh and I'd drive her car back to Minnesota. Linda agreed that she would stay in California a couple of extra weeks after Angie came home, to make moving arrangements and pack. The last several months had been a whirlwind and the next month or two would be the same.

The planning for the party and for the move back to Minnesota made the next two weeks pass quickly. When the day came to fly to California for the big surprise, Linda's mom and aunt were so excited. With Josh's help, everything fell into place perfectly.

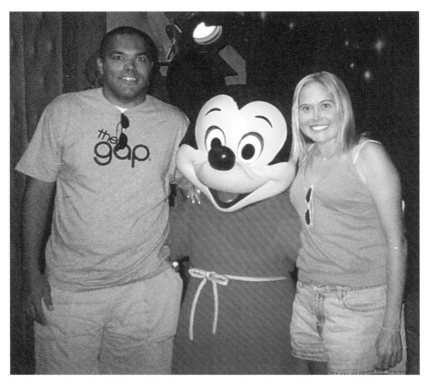

Josh arrived in La Jolla a few days early so that he and Angie could visit with Mickey.

Upon our arrival at the San Diego airport, I went to the baggage claim area to meet Linda and Angie. Bernelda and Sister Dorothy waited a minute or two before casually walking toward us at baggage claim. Linda was so surprised and happy; tears flowed. Angie had a huge smile. Josh had stayed at the apartment, decorating the place and later picking up the cake. He joined us at a restaurant for lunch before we all went to the apartment for birthday cake and conversation.

From Thursday through Sunday, we toured San Diego with our guests and took a drive up to Laguna Beach to share our special vacation locale with the ladies. We ate dinner by the ocean each night and thoroughly enjoyed our time together. Bernelda and Sister Dorothy returned to Minnesota on Sunday, Angie and Josh left the following Tuesday, and I departed by car two days later. Linda remained, as planned, to take care of the final details.

I spent most of my three-day drive home to Minnesota contemplating Angie's condition. She had a terrible cough by the time she and Josh had left for home. Based on the severity of her cough, I figured it might be time for another tune-up. We had already scheduled an appointment for her at the University of Minnesota CF Center for the following week.

I was concerned, of course, about Angela's pulmonary issues, but also worried that she might be suffering emotionally, feeling she had somehow failed to make a go of the big move to the West Coast. The reality of living near the ocean in California had not lived up to the exciting dream. I sensed Angela felt great disappointment that her health had let her down. I feared that the harsh threats and limitations of cystic fibrosis had pierced my daughter's spirit in a way I'd not seen before.

Arriving back in Minneapolis on Saturday, I accompanied Angie and Josh to a Neil Diamond concert that evening in St. Paul. Angie was much less tense, and happy to be back home with Josh. But she was holding her side and still had a bad cough. The results of the doctor's visit the next week did lead to a tune-up hospitalization for Angie and, for Linda, a premature return from California. The final packing and move had to wait for a while.

Knowing she had a date with him the night before she was going into the hospital, I asked Angie, "What about Josh?"

Though Angela had shared with Josh that she had cystic fibrosis, she had downplayed the seriousness and stressed that she was doing well. We would have trouble keeping him in the dark now that they had become so close. He'd surely worry about her if he didn't know where she was for a week or more. Angela saw the sense in telling Josh about her tune-up, but I could see she felt uncomfortable about tackling the conversation. I asked if she wanted me to talk to him. Angela readily agreed.

According to plan, Josh arrived for the date, and Angie stayed upstairs "getting ready" while he and I went downstairs to talk in the family room. Josh and I sat across from each other on the L-shaped sectional couch. I started by asking Josh what he already understood about cystic fibrosis from talking to Angie. He said he knew some but he wanted to know more. I tried to assure him that she was doing relatively well under the circumstances. I described the anatomical aspects of the disease and the nature of a tune-up, explaining to him that, for a week for two, Angie's lungs needed extra assistance and IV antibiotics to fight infection. We both focused on the positive aspects of the situation. We spoke generally about promising gene therapy and how life expectancy for people with cystic fibrosis was now thought to reach into the 30s and 40s.

I did not sense, even for one moment, that the seriousness of Angela's disease caused Josh to back away from her in any way. He visited her every other night while she was in the hospital. He usually showed up later in the evening just as Linda and I were leaving. Now that Josh was more aware of Angie's health challenges, our time with him, including vacations, would be easier. We could talk openly about planning and fitting therapies into the schedule.

Angie recovered quickly after this tune-up. The pseudomonas had not disappeared but was under control for the time being.

EARLY ON A SUNDAY MORNING, November 11, 2001, I received a call from my cousin Pat. Pat worked at the assisted-living facility where my eighty-year-old mother had been living for the past eighteen months in my hometown of Princeton, Minnesota. The call was to tell me that my mother, Elenora, was experiencing heart failure and had been taken to the nearby hospital. My sister, Joan, had gone to northern Minnesota and was not yet reachable by phone, and my half-brother Dennis lived in Michigan. I immediately drove the hour north to Princeton. I wasn't sure when I would return, or under what circumstances, so Linda and Angie remained at home awaiting updates. Angie's tune-up had done its job, but she still had a PICC line under her arm and she needed IV injections every four hours day and night. Linda had to do the injections while I was gone.

When I arrived at the hospital, I was told that Mom was in critical condition, and she might not survive the day. By late afternoon, however, she was cognizant and resting comfortably. We sat together and talked about many things. I mostly just wanted to be with her.

I kept my brother informed by phone and I finally reached Joan. She was on her way home to Princeton and due at the hospital around 8:30 P.M. Joan, who is a nurse, would be our mother's caregiver for the evening. Mom still seemed to be doing well around 6:30 P.M. At her urging, I agreed to return to Eden Prairie for the night and come back the next day after helping Linda with Angie's morning antibiotic injection.

Just before I left that evening, my mother looked at me with great seriousness and said, "I am so worried about Angie." My heart ached as I saw the sincerity and fear in her eyes. After fighting for her own life throughout the day, my dear mother was more concerned about her granddaughter. I tried to assure her, promising I would take care of Angela to the best of my ability. I urged Mom to focus on herself right now.

When I was ready to leave, I kissed my mother, told her I loved her and said I'd see her the following day. The drive back to Eden Prairie was a long and difficult one. I was still conflicted between staying overnight or going home to help Linda take care of Angela. I kept reminding myself that my sister was there; my mother was in good hands.

Around 6:30 the next morning, I received a call from Joan. Our mother had just passed away. Her heart had suddenly stopped. My sister and I cried together on the phone.

Our mother had endured great loss in her life. She lost her father when she was a child. Then, when her first husband died in a tractor accident, she had to sell the family farm. She bought a small house in town, took in tenants, and did sewing and laundry for others to pay the bills. Her second husband died soon after the horrific and untimely death of her young son.

As I drove back to Princeton to be with my sister, I thought again about everything my mother had endured. I thought about her concern for Angela. Had she had a premonition or was she just expressing her deepest worry that final night?

During the days following Mother's passing, we commuted between our home in Eden Prairie and my mother's home in Princeton, scheduling these travels around Angela's multiple daily therapies and antibiotics injections. Funeral arrangements were made and family business was completed.

Angela remained diligent about her health care despite sadness over the loss of her grandmother. Grandma's death was Angie's first experience with the loss of someone she loved. She and my mother had been very close. Angela had enjoyed Mom's perspective on life. Being from small-town America, my mother always knew the local gossip, and she and Angie often talked and laughed together. Mom's cooking was the best, particularly her turkey dinners on holidays. Recalling her wonderful cooking was particularly poignant with Thanksgiving only a couple of weeks away.

After Mother's wake, our family went to a restaurant for dinner. Angela needed an antibiotic injection prior to our drive home so we planned to stop back at Mother's apartment after our meal. However, when we got there at 11:00 P.M., the security system for the building was activated and we had no access. Fortunately, the night was not particularly cold for November in Minnesota. I looked at the dimly lit sitting area outside the main entrance. Angela's injection had to be done. We sat on the bench and did the procedure right there, but I felt frustrated that this horrible disease required such actions during our time of loss. I also thought about the explanation that might be required if the police happened by at that moment. We, no doubt, made a suspicious sight, appearing to inject drugs into a young girl's arm outside a barely lit building at night. The image was certainly one I'll not forget.

The next day, as we left the cemetery after my mother's interment, Angela made a comment that hit me like a punch to my gut. As we walked together, she mentioned to Linda and me that she never wanted to be buried underground. My heart hurt to realize that my beautiful twenty-year-old daughter was thinking about her own death. Even though people with cystic fibrosis are inclined to think about their own mortality at an early age, I had always hoped Angela could imagine herself enjoying a long life. Neither Linda nor I said anything that day, but we would have to honor Angela's direction when the time came.

Our family had a somber Thanksgiving. Angie eventually completed the course of antibiotics and the PICC line was removed from her arm. She had a little continued pain in her left chest area but, in general, seemed to be feeling well enough to continue with her interior design studies and work on her part-time eBay business. By then, Josh's own eBay business was fully established, as was his friendly online American Doll sales competition with Angie.

ON THE SATURDAY AFTER THANKSGIVING, Linda and I were in California, finalizing the details of vacating the apartment in La Jolla. While there, I took Linda to see Neil Diamond. The concert was part of the same tour as the concert I had enjoyed with Angela and Josh only weeks before. We were out late that night so we turned off the phone so we could sleep later the next morning. When we finally listened to voicemail messages, we heard Angie's cheerful shout as she asked, "Where is everybody?" She went on to say she had exciting news she wanted to share. Puppies! She had located a place with three female Maltese puppies.

Angie adopted a little white Maltese and named her Torrance, which meant spending more evenings at Josh's apartment. She took good care of Torrance, taking her for walks and ensuring her veterinary care. The new puppy added some much-needed extra cheer to the holiday season in 2001.

The year ended with us planning the best way to celebrate Angela's twenty-first birthday in March. We decided Las Vegas was a fitting locale for the big celebration. We made plans to stay for a week at the Venetian Hotel. Josh would join us and stay a couple of blocks away at the Riviera Hotel.

IT WAS A CELEBRATION TO REMEMBER. We had a wonderful time hanging out in Las Vegas, going to comedy shows and

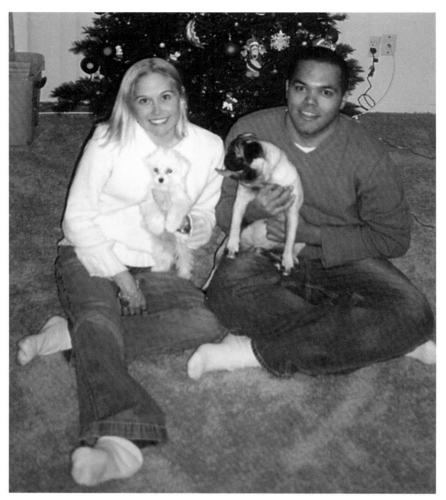

Angie, Torrance, Beyonce and Josh

concerts. Don Rickles was terrific. Linda and Angie did plenty of shopping. Josh and I did some gambling. Josh enjoyed sports betting. He was typically laid back and relaxed, except when he was involved in sports or sports-related activities. I liked that about him.

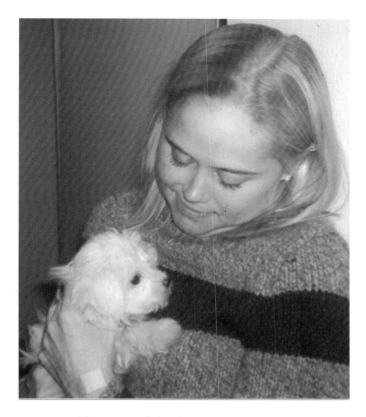

Torrance and Angie

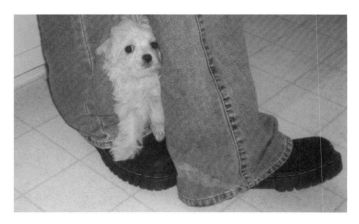

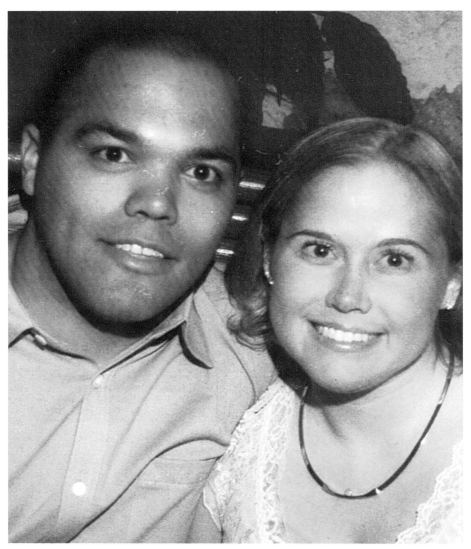

21ˢᵗ Birthday

The night of Angie's birthday, she dressed up. She wore a beautiful medium-length beige dress covered with lace. With her blonde hair in a stylish short cut, she looked absolutely radiant. Josh appeared a proud escort. We sat in a round corner booth at Kokomo's restaurant at the Mirage Hotel. We each ordered our favorite meal, and I walked away knowing the dinner had been worth every penny. Now we were on to the gambling tables.

Angela played slots for a while, some video poker games, and a few games of blackjack. I expected to spend several hours "donating" our funds alongside Angie on her first night of legal gambling. But Angela announced she'd had enough after about forty-five minutes. When asked why, she said gambling seemed an overrated waste of time; she preferred to spend her available dollars shopping. (I knew she was smart!) She was also wise in that she refrained from drinking alcohol that night. My responsible twenty-one-year-old daughter knew alcohol was detrimental to her health, would impair her concentration during her therapy, and the taste was not worth the potential harm. We ended the night with a pleasant gondola ride at the Venetian Hotel.

PART THREE

WHATEVER
IT
TAKES

ANGELA BEGAN A HEAVY REGIMEN of a drug called prednisone in the spring. Prednisone is an anti-inflamma-
tory steroid that initially provided some relief from the
chest pain Angela had been feeling on the left chest wall. The
pain in her side was not initially diagnosed, but tests finally determined the cause to be pleurisy resulting from the pseudomonas
bacteria. Bacteria had migrated from her lungs to irritate the
chest wall. Prednisone is often called a miracle drug, due to its
effectiveness. However, continued heavy doses can also result in
significant long-term side effects such as calcium reduction and
osteoporosis. We were told to watch carefully for certain things,
such as puffiness in Angie's face, irritability, or mood swings.

In April, Torrance was due to be spayed. Angie asked if her dog could recover at our house. I agreed despite my allergies and, even before I had time to develop an allergic reaction, I, too, fell in love with Torrance. I began taking special allergy medication so Torrance could continue to live with us.

Otherwise, the spring and early summer were routine and tranquil. Angie was on a schedule of three to four therapies per day but still found time for Josh, Torrance, her studies, shopping, and hanging out with Linda and me. We ate our regular dinners at our favorite restaurants. Weeks seemed to pass quickly when Angie's health seemed to be going well. Although we could see that Angie was not feeling terrific, we believed that, if we remained diligent about her therapies and medications, her health would eventually improve.

ANGIE HEARD ABOUT an American Girl doll warehouse sale in July in Madison, Wisconsin. She convinced Linda to go with her on the secret two-day "shopping trip" to Madison, but she didn't mention it to Josh. At the sale Angie loaded up on inventory at significant discounts. Linda and I were amused to observe her competitiveness with Josh. I teased Angie for keeping her excursion a secret, and I told her Josh would have appreciated her ingenuity.

Josh was busy with other entrepreneurial endeavors as well. The owner of the Domino's pizza where Josh worked sold the franchise to purchase a Quizno's Sub store and hired Josh to be his manager. This was a good promotion. Josh and I talked often about the business. Observing his management skills, I was impressed. I offered to help him acquire the Quizno's franchise from the current owner if ever the opportunity arose.

During August of 2002, Josh joined us in Laguna Beach for the first half of our annual vacation. He stayed at a nearby hotel. Angie preferred this arrangement, as she wanted her privacy when the time came to do therapies and take her daily medications. Understanding her required regimen, Josh respectfully gave Angie the space she needed for her care to be completed.

One evening we ate at Angela's favorite restaurant at a table overlooking the ocean in La Jolla. I was tickled when she ordered the most enormous lobster, then amazed that my tiny-framed daughter had the appetite and capacity to devour a lobster that size. After dinner the four of us attended an Alicia Keys concert. Angie loved music and when she had a favorite artist or group she followed their career thoroughly. From her childhood concerts with New Kids on the Block and Boyz to Men, to Christina Aguilera and many others, Angie enjoyed being a fan and quickly knew every song the artist sang. This was also the case with her love of Alicia Keys. Angela bought tickets online for the concert, which was to be staged on a pier in the San Diego Harbor. We revived our NBA scalping talents the night of the concert and "upgraded" to perfect seats in the third row. The sun set over the harbor just as the show began. We had an enchanted evening.

We enjoyed ten days together at the Surf and Sand Hotel. Angie and I still took our nighttime walks on the beach. In recent years, and now with Josh on vacation with us, we had made these walks a little less frequently, but I treasured each one. The waves were mesmerizing on our last night. We stood on our deck overlooking the surf only a few feet below. The stars were shining and airplane lights occasionally flashed through the night sky over the ocean. Catalina Island became invisible after a majestic sunset. I put my arms around my daughter, and we stood still in a hug for several moments.

By SEPTEMBER THE PAIN in Angie's left chest wall intensified. She sometimes folded her left arm to press the back of her left hand against her chest. This kind of pressure helped some. Angie looked like she had a wing when she held that position. Seeing her do that was always a clear sign to Linda and me that chest pain was bothering her.

At the same time, Angela was beginning to experience some side effects from the prednisone. She was referred to an endocrinologist who advised quarterly intravenous injections of calcium. X-rays had shown that Angie had developed small hairline fractures in her spine, a possible side effect of the drug in combination with harsh coughing. She was not experiencing any discomfort in her back—at least, no pain she considered significant relative to the other daily aches, pains, and discomforts that come with cystic fibrosis.

Her first calcium injection was in late September 2002. The continued use of prednisone was prescribed despite the side effects. I believe Angela was having a difficult emotional time. She knew she was going to have to add quarterly calcium injections to her already demanding medical care regimen, and she was continually uncomfortable because of the chest pain.

Linda and I tried to think of ways to help Angie fight the negative effects of the medication. We were ready and willing to do whatever was necessary to help build back her endurance. We made a family commitment. We'd each get into better shape. We could build a gym in our house and work out together. We'd hire a trainer; follow a regimen.

But Angie was tired so much of the time. Taking Torrance for walks was the most physical exertion she could handle. Her little companion lay across Angie's lap while she worked at the computer to handle her eBay business. Filling five to ten orders a day left her with little energy to see Josh after he finished work. Without giving him much explanation, Angie often told him not to come over. She cancelled plans sometimes at the last minute. Angie told Josh on the day of a friend's wedding that her knee hurt and she could not go with him. He was angry, saying he didn't even know anyone else going to the wedding. She made him an apology card and wrote her promise to make it up to him. But the cancellations continued. For Josh to know she had cystic fibrosis and be aware of the therapies and daily cares was not a problem, but for Josh to see her feeling so poorly was not acceptable to Angie. She now wanted privacy.

Josh and Angie finally agreed to "take a break." She made him promise they would still be best friends and still go on a planned trip to Las Vegas together at Christmas. He readily agreed; he didn't want to lose Angie. The two maintained contact but stopped going out. During all that time, Josh did not realize that CF was responsible for the change in their relationship.

ANGELA'S CHEST PAIN seemed to be getting worse, and the prednisone, and then Vioxx, dosages continued to increase. Another hospitalization was imminent—just another tune-up, we hoped. By early October the pain in Angie's side was constant; the drugs were providing less and less relief. She was seen at the CF Center, and we learned that the level of pseudomonas in her pulmonary tests had increased. Only a year before, Dr. Eddy had commented that Angie's lungs looked as healthy as a "normal" person's!

On October 11, 2002, she was admitted to the University Hospital for a one-week stay. During this tune-up hospitalization, Dr. Eddy decided to reduce and eventually try to eliminate Angie's use of prednisone. The alternative plan was to use a combination of opiates and other drugs. Linda and

Angela listened as I questioned Dr. Eddy about the side effects of this medication regimen that included narcotic drugs instead of prednisone. Rather than providing a detailed explanation about his course of action, the doctor assured us that the side effects of this combination were less harmful than continuing to use prednisone. Although we did not have a full understanding of the consequences of taking narcotics at this point, we were desperate for solutions and relief for Angie.

In the hospital she was given the usual intravenous antibiotics, along with the new medicines and the prednisone. Weaning off the prednisone was to occur at home over the following weeks. We assumed a successful tune-up would bring the infection under control, Angela's lung function would improve, and her pain would be reduced. Linda and I also hoped the tune-up would restore Angela's health to the level she enjoyed months earlier. We hoped she'd have less need for the narcotics once she was released from the hospital.

Prior to the hospitalization, Angie told Josh she was leaving town to visit her sick uncle in the hospital. But after she was out of contact for several days, and he received no answer calling her cell phone, Josh called our house and left a message on the machine. When Angie learned that he'd called the house, she was irritated and told him not to do that again.

Angie came home with a PICC line and antibiotics, as well as the new medications. A gradual reduction in prednisone began. Her PICC line was removed at a clinic appointment on November 8th, and she was feeling better. But just days later, Angela began to experience severe bowel pains, bloating, and vomiting. Linda called the CF Center that Monday morning to report the new symptoms. A prescription for a mild laxative was called in to our pharmacy. The laxative had no immediate effect. Angie couldn't eat; she experienced reflux and more vomiting.

Linda called the CF Center again Tuesday morning. This time, the nurse suggested that Angela drink Mucomyst—the medication used in making the aerosol Angela inhaled while doing the chest therapies. We were told that drinking Mucomyst might break up the mucus that was likely causing an intestinal blockage. As instructed, Angela tried this strategy through the day without results. She discovered the taste of Mucomyst was less repulsive if chilled, so we prepared the medicine over ice—but still no results. Angie's discomfort was intensifying. Linda and I were deeply concerned.

When Linda called the CF Center on Wednesday morning, November 13, we were finally told to bring Angela to the emergency room. I left my office immediately and drove the fifteen to twenty minutes to our home. I felt so sorry that Angie had to go to the hospital again. I prayed this crisis could be solved within an evening or a day. After all, constipation wasn't a life-threatening condition in the world of modern medical technology—was it?

At home, I found Angie packing items in anticipation of a hospital stay that might be longer than a matter of hours. She had the clothes she liked to wear around the hospital, usually a T-shirt or sweatshirt, shorts or sweatpants, open-toed sandals, and heavy socks in case the room was cold. She brought her laptop computer so she could stay connected to friends via the Internet. She always had a book or two. This time she was reading *Fighting Back* by Bill Sammon, about America's response to 9/11. Finally, she packed a couple of stuffed animals that gave her a degree of comfort during those lonely and, often, sleepless nights in the hospital.

I loaded the car. Angie was uncomfortable and bloated. She never before had any extra weight on her tiny frame, so the bloating over the last few days was noticeable. She was lethargic from the narcotic medications, but she said goodbye to Torrance and was able to walk to the car and climb in. As we arrived at the emergency room entrance, Angie stepped out of her sandals and put on tennis shoes. She left her sandals and her mittens on the floor in the back of my car.

So, into the emergency room we went. We might as well have been entering a torture chamber on a different planet.

ALL THAT'S REQUIRED

Once Angie was admitted to the University Hospital emergency room on Wednesday, we were anxious to meet the pulmonologist on call. We learned that the CF Center physicians were out of town at a cystic fibrosis convention. As Angie lay on the exam table, Linda and I sat, stood and paced during the long wait for the pulmonologist. Nurses and others came in and out, checking on Angie. When the physician finally arrived, she confirmed that pulmonologists from the CF Center were not due back from the convention in Seattle until late Friday. She said she usually worked at a different hospital in Minneapolis. I asked if she was a CF specialist, and she assured us she had experience with "chronic illness."

Linda and I were immediately concerned. Dr. Warwick had often told us a doctor needed to care for at least sixty to seventy CF patients to have a comprehensive understanding of the disease and its complexities. I asked more questions, and Linda asked a few too. In most cases, Angie waited until after the doctors left the room to express her concerns, but this day she was feeling too miserable to say much.

She was taken to the radiology department for x-rays of her abdomen. The pulmonologist told us the x-rays showed that Angie had a significant-sized intestinal blockage. Reviewing Angie's medications, the physician expressed surprise, saying, "I can't believe she's been on these narcotics for a month without being prescribed a stool softener!"

The doctor explained that "normally" a stool softener is prescribed when a patient is taking narcotics for any extended period. She made a note in Angie's chart about the absence of stool softener. This was a new worry for Angie, Linda, and me. We had not been aware of that potential side effect.

The course of treatment for the blockage was to be a series of enemas and the administration of an electrolyte solution called Golytely through a nasogastric tube (NG tube). This laxative liquid was to flow through the digestive system, cleansing and hopefully pushing through whatever was blocking the intestine. The plastic NG tube was to go into Angela's nose and down into her stomach. After the physician left the room, Angie commented in anger, "I can't believe Dr. Eddy did this to me!"

When Angie saw Dr. Eddy five days earlier for an examination and the removal of her PICC line, he had not expressed concern about any aspect of Angie's current medications. She had hoped she was on the healing side of the equation. But since

Sunday, her spirits had faded and now her face looked so sad—a resigned, "Here we go again, but this is even worse," expression.

Angie was finally transferred from the emergency room to an assigned patient room. Most of the patients on her floor had cancer, and many were on narcotic medications for pain. Angie heard again and again from her nurses that she should have been given stool softeners from the start, especially because she was on high dosages of drugs that "naturally" caused constipation.

Several different respiratory service clinicians tried without success to insert an NG tube through Angie's nose. She tried to cooperate with their efforts to push the tube in her nose, but she winced and cried out, and soon had a bloody nose. She was given a morphine pump to manage her abdominal pain.

I did not trust that these people understood the everyday aspects of CF. As clinicians continued to struggle to insert the tube, Linda and I each explained to the doctor about some of the factors that might be causing their difficulty with inserting the NG tube—that Angie's nasal passages had often been inflamed due to allergies, and her sinus surgery two years earlier had left scarring. But the doctor did not appear interested in the added information. Angie's annoyance at the situation was obvious. Despite the ongoing inability to insert an NG tube, the pulmonologist insisted that things were "under control." The more she said that, the less I believed her. Watching Angie's misery, I commented, "You must have a better technique than jamming this tube up her nose."

One of the respiratory clinicians responded by suggesting a pediatric NG tube. They were smaller and could usually be inserted easily, using a small amount of sedation. The current procedure had to be stopped anyway because Angie's nose was now bleeding profusely. I asked the pulmonologist if she could try the pediatric NG tube alternative. She said inserting a pediatric NG tube couldn't be done right away because the needed sedation was not possible in a patient room. That procedure had to be done on a different floor of the hospital. The doctor left, saying she'd "look into it."

Through the rest of the day and evening, Angela endured several uncomfortable gastric enemas to cleanse the large intestine. The process was messy, embarrassing and frustrating for Angie. At one point on the way to the bathroom she slipped on the wet floor. Our stress was building. Linda cried angry tears, watching our daughter's misery without being able to help.

That evening I asked the pulmonologist if any CF specialist could see Angie. We were told none were available. How could this be? Wasn't this place a major CF center? I asked if a gastrointestinal (GI) consult had been requested—could a GI specialist examine Angie? The pulmonologist said she was "quite capable" of following protocol and, "that's all that is required at the moment."

On Thursday morning, November 14, the NG tube had still not been placed. When the pulmonologist arrived that day, we again asked her about using a pediatric NG tube with mild sedation. Though I thought she appeared reluctant, she arranged for the procedure to be done later that afternoon. I was with Angie as the NG tube was placed. She was relaxed and sleepy from the sedating medication. The placement was done easily in moments.

The Golytely was begun by 4:30 P.M., but Angie was now extremely frustrated and in great discomfort. The morphine was only helping a little. She hated the feeling of the tube in her nose and down her throat, and she still had the pain in her stomach. She wanted to pull out the tubing. I told her in a comforting voice, "You can't do that. We have to get you better."

Linda rubbed Angie's feet and tried to divert her attention from her discomfort, talking about *All My Children* and Torrance's antics.

We made a formal request for a GI specialist to be consulted, but again the pulmonologist insisted she had the training and experience to handle the situation. Linda and I remained doubtful. Hour by hour Angela's stomach was filled with Golytely. She was experiencing more and more breathing difficulty as a result of bloating. Her oxygen saturation was low so she was given a nasal cannula with oxygen. She had to sit up. Watching our daughter endure so much continuing discomfort was heart wrenching. To our beautiful, intelligent, and proud young daughter, the procedures felt degrading and embarrassing, as well as painful.

I took a break from Angie's bedside to call Barb, Angela's nurse at the CF Center. She had known our family since Angela was a baby. I told her our concerns about the pulmonologist caring for Angie. I said we questioned the doctor's experience and competence. Barb tried to assure me that the pulmonologist was following protocol and speaking by phone with Dr. Eddy. She reminded us that Dr. Eddy and the other CF doctors were returning from Seattle late the following evening.

The rest of Thursday evening was spent watching Angela receive Golytely for four hours straight with no successful outcome. We filled the time watching television, helping Angie do respiratory therapies and helping her shift positions—from sitting, lying, or side to side.

Linda or I, or both of us, were committed to being with Angie at all times. Continuing to do bronchial drainage therapies was especially important during any medical crisis. Those were the times when regular treatments for patients with CF were easy to overlook. So, mixed in with everything else, we made sure Angie did six thirty-minute bronchial drainage therapies each day. We took breaks, one of us at a time, to grab food from the hospital cafeteria. Angie had not eaten since Sunday and her abdomen continued to bloat.

When the pulmonologist checked on Angie late that night, I asked, "Is it appropriate for Angie to have a CT scan to find out more about the location and nature of the blockage?"

The doctor explained that the current course of treatment would not change with any information from a CT scan. Her plan was to administer more Golytely the next day. She informed us that nurses had not used sufficient volumes of Golytely that day.

For the second night, I dozed on the windowsill to be on hand if Angie needed anything; she was groggy from the morphine. Linda went home to feed and let out Torrance. I helped Angie to and from the bathroom many times in the night, negotiating the IV poles and tubing.

By the next day, Friday, Linda and I felt so vulnerable for our daughter. At one point Angie opened her eyes, looked down at her legs, and asked in a whimper, "Why are my legs swollen?" Edema had developed from fluid retention.

I wanted to rescue my daughter. I wished I could take her place. On high doses of morphine that day, Angie became hallucinatory. She was saying some hilarious things in her stupor, but Linda and I were more frightened than entertained. We found no humor in any part of what was happening. I made another call to Barb, expressing our strong desire for another doctor to review Angie's care and examine her. We were convinced this pulmonologist was in over her head. She was still unwilling to call in a GI specialist, and she continued to refuse to do a CT scan. After hearing how poorly Angie was doing, Barb now expressed alarm. She promised to call Dr. Eddy to see what could be done. But we didn't hear back from her that day.

Angela's situation continued to worsen through the day. The Golytely was administered again for several hours. Still nothing. With so much fluid pressure on Angie's diaphragm, she was having trouble catching her breath. She was terribly bloated and the fluid in her stomach was causing the lower lobes of her lungs to collapse—a concern to any CF patient. Her oxygen had to be turned up quite a bit to stop her from passing out. When she began to gurgle in her sleep, I called in the resident and told him, "This is not working!"

The Golytely was finally terminated at 3:00 A.M. Angie was now awake and aware of the situation. After so many precarious hours, she said, "Dad, what can we do? I feel like I'm not getting better."

I was crazed with frustration, desperate to find help for Angie. Her pulmonological health was deteriorating rapidly;

she was feeling worse in every other way as well. The CF doctors were back in town and were scheduled to hold their annual CF Family Conference during the day on Saturday at the University Radisson Hotel, only two blocks from the hospital. Dr. Eddy and the other CF doctors would be in attendance. Linda was going home for the night to care for Torrance. I asked her to be back by 9:00 A.M. I was going to the conference in the morning to plead for help.

Three days earlier, Angela had walked into an emergency room with "constipation" or "a bowel obstruction." Now she appeared to be in critical condition. Linda and I were afraid Angie might die; now she was scared, too. I had tried not to convey the extent of our fear to Angie but we could each see that her medical care was not being delivered with any sense of urgency. I hoped Dr. Eddy would change all that on Saturday.

ABOUT 10:00 SATURDAY MORNING, November 16, I walked the two blocks to the University Radisson Hotel where the CF Family Conference was being held. I had inquired and been told this was the time for a scheduled mid-morning break. I had prepared a list of Angela's symptoms I hoped would adequately demonstrate her desperate condition: her inability to maintain sufficient oxygen saturation in her blood with room air only, her severe bloating, edema in her legs, and her growing loss of hope.

The room was crowded when I arrived at the conference, but I saw Dr. Warwick almost immediately. He was focused on socializing with conference attendees and did not appear to grasp the seriousness of what I was telling him. He suggested Angela might have some vitamin deficiency and returned to his conversation with colleagues. I was furious and crushed. He was too distracted by the conference to focus on my child's crisis. I quickly moved on and sought out Dr. Eddy.

I found the CF nurse, Barb, sitting behind a family information table. She did not apologize or provide any excuse for not getting back to me as she had promised the day before. I shared with her my list of concerns. Amid tears, I pleaded with her to have Dr. Eddy visit and examine Angela. Barb said Dr. Eddy was preparing his presentation for that afternoon, but she assured me she would tell him about my request and my concerns. She was "certain" Dr. Eddy would want to visit Angie as soon as possible. I thanked her and went back to the hospital.

Angie, Linda, and I waited in desperation all afternoon and evening for Dr. Eddy. During that time, Angie finally received a GI consult. Though the physician did not speak to us, he changed Angie's treatment. No Golytely or any other medications were being used at this point to clear the blockage. Instead, the process was reversed to extract the Golytely; the NG tube was being used now to suction fluids out of her stomach. As hours passed and Dr. Eddy did not arrive or contact us, my fear and rage were building. I could not believe he would not come to the hospital, just two blocks away, after my plea to Barb. But, surely we would see him Sunday morning.

Linda stayed with Angela, and I went home to take care of Torrance, shower and try to sleep. I came back early in the morning to be in Angie's room when Dr. Eddy came. But Sunday morning came and went without a visit from Dr. Eddy.

Despite continued suctioning, Angela's breathing was more labored by the hour. She had gained at least twenty pounds of fluid weight since Wednesday.

Linda stayed with Angela while I left the hospital on Sunday afternoon to stop at my office. On the way I decided to try to obtain Dr. Eddy's home number from directory assistance. His home number was listed, and he answered the phone. He explained that he had discussed Angie's condition the day before with the pulmonologist who was treating Angie. He didn't feel that examining her personally was "necessary." In a firm but polite voice I told him, "I strongly disagree." When I shared with him the list of concerning symptoms, he admitted that the situation sounded "troublesome." He said he'd try to visit Angie that afternoon.

Despite being on so much morphine for her discomfort, Angie was aware of her condition. She had heard the pulmonologist describe the lack of prescribed stool softeners to go along with the narcotics as "bad medicine." She had heard the same from several of the floor nurses. She knew of our unanswered requests for a CT scan and an earlier GI consult. This was the fifth day in the hospital, and Angie was no better than when she first arrived—she felt far worse. Angela now used some justified expletives to describe how furious she was with Dr. Eddy, who never did show up on Sunday. Linda and I were angry too. Though we were certain Dr. Eddy would come in on Monday morning, Angie now said she wanted nothing to do with him.

When Angie and I were alone on Sunday night we talked about how to proceed from here. I had no doubt surgery was likely needed to remove the intestinal blockage. Surgery should have already been done days ago. We discussed alternatives for her care. We considered seeking out a different doctor or a different hospital, but that would mean a great deal of change and getting a new group of people up to speed about Angie and her condition. After reviewing our alternatives and knowing surgery was needed soon, we both felt the situation was too critical to risk losing more time before she was treated. Angie decided to give Dr. Eddy another chance.

Dr. Eddy came to see Angela at about nine o'clock Monday morning. After a brief examination he determined that surgery was the only solution to the intestinal blockage. Everything else had been tried.

SURGERY FOR A CF PATIENT is always a risk because of the need for a respirator. Linda and I prayed that no irreparable damage had been done to Angie's lungs during the past five days. Dr. Eddy talked to Angie about performing a bronchoscopy while she was sedated for surgery. He could inspect her lungs and remove any foreign material. This procedure could possibly improve her lung function. That sounded promising. Could we be on the road to ending this nightmare after days of suffering and trauma for our precious daughter? After the surgery and recovery, would Angie finally be able to resume her life?

The rest of Monday was filled with tests, including the CT scan, and meetings with a GI specialist and the surgeon. Late in the day we discovered that the surgery could not be scheduled with the right doctor, at the right time, in the right operating room, until the following day. Linda and I were aggravated by the delay; other treatment options had been exhausted several days earlier. Angie was in pain; her pulmonary condition had deteriorated more each day, as had her spirits. And now surgery was delayed yet another day.

I stayed the night with Angie. Neither of us slept much; we were both anxious. At one point during the night, I opened my eyes to see her sitting up in bed, watching me as I rested in a chair. I smiled and we talked some.

Angie said, "Daddy is such a good sport."

I looked into her eyes and said, "Angie, it's so easy to be a good sport when I am caring for the person I love more than anything in the world."

Angie only said, "I love you, too."

Calling me a good sport was her way of saying thanks for being at her side during the experience, helping her navigate pain and personal degradation with as much dignity as possible. I was awash with love for my daughter.

Activity in Angie's room picked up substantially the next morning. Preparation for surgery on Tuesday included two bronchial therapy treatments before 10:00 A.M. Doctors came in and out of her room; surgery was to occur around noon.

During the second bronchial treatment Angie sat in a chair while Linda and I sat on the bed, taking turns holding the aerosol mask. Angela was too weak to hold the mask to her face. We adjusted the air pressures periodically as needed on the therapy machine.

Angie looked up and said in a soft voice, "I'm scared."

My heart sank, and my eyes welled up. I leaned over to Angie, touching her forehead squarely with my own and told her, "Angie, it's okay to be afraid, but know that you have great doctors taking care of you, and you are at one of the best hospitals in America. In a few days you'll be on the road to recovery. Your mom and I love you and will take care of you." I didn't know what else to say. Angie saw the tears in my eyes.

About 11:00 A.M., Linda and I escorted Angie down the hall to the pre-surgery waiting area. We each hugged her and told her we loved her. We passed the time talking about our next trip. Our plan was to go to Las Vegas in December. Now we'd go as soon as Angie was feeling well enough. I added, "Josh can come along again."

Angie smiled and said, "I'd really like that."

Finally, everyone and everything was ready for her. Angela was wheeled down the hall sitting upright on a gurney because she was too uncomfortable to lie on her back. As she passed through the double doors leading to the operating room, Linda and I told her again and again how much we loved her. Then we were left with our hopes and prayers. Surely nothing could be worse than the past six days.

But we soon learned that it could.

AFTER SEVERAL HOURS OF WAITING, Linda and I received word that the abdominal surgery to clear Angie's small intestine was successful. A six-pound blockage was removed. The surgeon explained that although the operation went well, a problem had developed with Angie's intubation and sedation. He said, "Her lungs had difficulty inflating on the respirator but she seems to be doing fine now." He assured us this was not uncommon for patients with cystic fibrosis.

Linda and I immediately went to see Angie in the surgical ICU on the fourth floor where she was still on a respirator. When she was finally conscious, she wrote notes, saying the respirator tubing was painful; she wanted it out "now." We each tried to assure her the ventilator was necessary for the moment but she would be all right. She just closed her eyes. The doctors increased her sedation so she could rest comfortably.

Once Angela was more comfortable and able to sleep in the ICU, Linda and I drove home, planning to return early the next morning. For the first time in six days, one of us did not stay at the hospital with Angie. I called the hospital to check on her before going to bed. The nurse said she was fine. Keeping the phone next to the bed, we collapsed in sleep, feeling relief that Angie was now on a three-to-five day recovery path.

Early the next morning, I called again to check on Angela. Her nurse was distressed, saying, "We had an awful night." He quickly explained that Angie had developed an infection and had become septic, requiring emergency intervention. The infection was in her bloodstream, which meant bacteria could travel to every organ in her body, including her lungs. During the night, surgeons had inserted a central line in her neck to more closely monitor her vitals in and around Angie's heart and lungs.

Linda and I rushed back to the hospital to be at Angie's side, hoping this was only a setback. We felt guilty for not being there. We were even more upset that the hospital staff had not called us during the night. Our daughter could have died! When we arrived at Angie's bedside, she looked the same as she had the night before, except for the new central line. We were given a grave assessment of her condition and prognosis. The ICU doctors told us that Angie's chances of survival were slim as a result of the sepsis. Her lungs were not likely to be able to fight the infection.

Linda and I could not believe what we were hearing. Reluctant to give up hope, we continued to ask questions, trying to get a comprehensive picture of Angie's status. Does everyone die from sepsis? The ICU doctors said clearly that Angie might not live through the day. Linda collapsed and was helped to a chair. One of the doctors gave her some medication to help her cope with the shock and grief. I was concerned for Linda. I could not imagine how she would survive the loss of her daughter, her constant companion, and our only child. She adored Angie as I did. I used every ounce of strength I could muster to not crash as well. If Angie had any chance of survival, I had to stay in control, pay close attention, and do what I could to monitor her care.

AFTER TWENTY-ONE YEARS OF FIGHTING this horrible disease quietly and alone, Linda and I now needed the aid and comfort of everyone. We would make a final all-inclusive stand against CF for our beloved daughter. I began making phone calls to family and friends.

AID
AND
COMFORT

inda's parents were the first family members to arrive along with Linda's sister Judi, brother Ron, and nieces, Tracy and Terry. My business partner and friend, Grant Lindaman, and his wife, Kathi, arrived within hours of my call and stayed by our side. Grant told me not to worry about work, to only focus on Angela and Linda.

Linda's mother took immediate charge of making certain every spiritual step was taken on Angela's behalf. Our priest from Pax Christi Catholic Church in Eden Prairie was asked to come to the hospital to perform the Anointing of the Sick—the sacrament formerly called Last Rites or Extreme Unction. Everything was happening so fast.

On November 21, 2002, as Fr. Tim prayed over Angela, our family and many of our friends surrounded her bed. The constant rhythm of the respirator reverberated through the room.

I thought, *If we are praying to an omnipotent God that could take this precious girl to a realm C.S. Lewis referred to as "inconceivable and unimaginable" for eternity, then the same God is also capable of delivering a miracle and saving Angie's life.* I decided to do everything I could do from the human side. I wanted Angie alive. I wanted her well again. I'd do anything, except watch her suffer unnecessarily. So Linda and I, along with the ICU medical staff and a great many devoted family and friends, began the crusade to save Angie.

Linda and I moved right into the fourth-floor waiting lounge. We had no idea how long we'd be staying, but we would be there for as long as necessary. The doctors referred to Angela's status as "hour-to-hour," which the nurses told us meant Angie could die at any moment.

Despite those initial grave predictions, Angie's condition improved slightly over the next few days, to the surprise of her doctors. But her condition remained "critical." The abdominal surgery, although successful, was also most likely the source of the sepsis infection. Angie was unconscious, under heavy sedation and still on the respirator. Every bodily function was being monitored. We were reminded daily by the doctors that she had little or no chance of survival. CF patients who are placed on a respirator for more than a day or two rarely get off the machine. Plus, Angela was fighting serious infections. Doctors occasionally inquired as to whether we wished to continue life support, but we could not give up on Angela. She was a fighter and, besides, unexplained miracles happen.

After each conversation about "letting Angie go," Linda and I tried to imagine what Angie might want us to do. We concluded that she loved life and would want to fight as long as possible. She had fought daily for each breath and for life itself. CF patients are fighters. Linda and I could not stop fighting until we thought Angie would.

I was blessed to have a best friend and business partner of twenty-seven years in my life. Grant and I had run our financial planning business together since shortly after college. We had an amazing professional staff and most of my clients had become my friends as well. Everyone was so loving and supportive. Grant and our office staff took complete charge of my day-to-day tasks. My clients repeatedly told me not to worry about them. I was touched by their heartfelt kindness.

I went into my office two or three times a week in the evening or on weekends so I could quickly finish what I needed to do without interruption. This allowed me to avoid seeing coworkers and having to discuss Angie's dire condition and the severity of the crisis. Those were hard conversations that I preferred to avoid. I took some work back to the hospital to do when I was alone with Angela.

Linda and I rented a hotel room near the hospital. We never did sleep there, but the room was a private place to shower and rest occasionally. We were in the fight of our lives; we had to be prepared in every possible way to carry on.

Angela's lungs were holding up, so far. Several antibiotics were fighting the infections. The nursing staff sat Angie up in a chair for a part of each day and reset the respirator occasionally so she, though unconscious, began to take her own breaths. The doctors' conversation began to take on a more hopeful tone: "This is going to be a long haul and a difficult task but recovery is possible and is slowly underway."

On November 26, one week after her surgery and a week since we had last spoken with Angela, we now hoped that within a few more days she might be conscious and on the road to recovery. Was a miracle occurring?

Linda and I remained continuous dwellers in the 4D lounge. The "Family Room" became our home. We ate, slept, worked, and met with doctors when we were not caring for Angie or talking with visitors. Other families came in and out of the lounge. Since Angie was in a surgical ICU, activity was constant and unpredictable. A continuing stream of strangers slept on couches, chairs, or on the floor near us. Getting rest was a challenge.

The 4D ICU was the place for the "sickest of the sick." The surgical ICU team members were true professionals. The six members of the physician team were specialists in facing and responding to critical patients. They were gentle and skilled at communicating with patients and families about difficult circumstances and choices. Their efforts to save Angela and cope with crisis after crisis were truly heroic.

MOST PATIENTS PASSED THROUGH 4D for only hours or days as they recovered from their critical status or surgery. Usually, patients were moved to regular patient floors before eventually going home. And some patients didn't survive their critical condition. But Angela was one of those rare patients who remained critical for much longer than days, and even longer than weeks. Her room and the 4D family lounge had become our world. That world took a sharp turn on Thursday, November 28, 2002, Thanksgiving. Our hopes for a quick recovery ended that day.

Around 10:00 A.M. Dr. Eddy came to examine Angela. He recommended another bronchoscopy to remove what appeared to be a mucous plug in the upper lobe of her left lung. Linda and I consented. The procedure was performed in Angela's room with the curtain pulled.

I could hear the conversation between Dr. Eddy and the assisting resident as they carried out the procedure. About ten minutes after they began, their work went in an unexpected direction. As the plug was removed, a blood clot broke open, causing massive bleeding throughout Angela's lungs. Immediately, Dr. Eddy summoned the on-call surgeon, who was at the nursing station only yards away. She literally came running. As she rushed passed me into Angie's room, she gave me a look I read as, "This is bad!" Linda and I listened from the other side of the curtain as another resident and a nurse raced in to help Angie.

Blood was spreading throughout Angie's lungs, filling her airways. Two drainage tubes were inserted. We were told the flowing blood was a "river" for infection to spread throughout her lungs. Blood loss was one concern, but worse was that Angela's blood-filled airways were already, or would soon become, unable to provide oxygen to her body or successfully remove carbon dioxide (CO_2) from her body. I learned quick-ly about pH levels and how the human body can become too acidic to sustain life, how organs then begin to shut down and the patient dies. The ICU doctor said, finally, that this was likely the end.

The next six hours were excruciating. Thanksgiving became a day seared into our minds as we stood by helplessly as one horror followed another. The force of air being pumped into Angie's lungs had to be elevated for oxygenation to occur. But the air had to be forced through blood-filled airways, and doing so blew holes right through Angela's lungs. Air was leaking from her lungs into her chest cavity. Additional chest tubes had to be inserted through her ribcage to withdraw the leaked air. Otherwise, air pressure in her chest cavity could force a lung to collapse. A total of eleven tubes were eventually inserted into Angie's chest. Linda and I were in shock; the ghastliness and horror of what was happening to our little girl was overwhelming. Our hopes were smashed. In our sadness and grief, we again summoned family and friends to the hospital.

Josh was shocked and distressed to learn how serious things had become. Angie's friend J.D. offered to take care of Torrance at his house for the duration. Josh and J.D. each made calls to other friends.

My friend Dick Johnson and his wife Jeanne came to our sides immediately. Dick spent four of the next eight nights at the hospital with us. He volunteered to stay in Angie's room and take notes of whatever happened so that I could take breaks to rest in the Family Room lounge. He kept a log of her blood gases and any other detail that occurred in the night. I was able to sleep for short periods, knowing Dick was keeping close watch.

Dick Johnson says…

My wife Jeanne and I were in San Diego on Thanksgiving when we called Don's cell phone to check in. No return call. Strange for Don not to call back. After another unreturned call, we checked with his office. Don's partner, Grant, told us Angela was in the hospital, not doing well. Jeanne and I returned to Minneapolis, dropped off our bags, and went directly to the hospital Intensive Care Unit. No words can describe the situation. Angela's life was hanging in the balance . . . my friends in anguish . . . I wanted to help. My professional training as a psychotherapist went out the window. All I could do, instinctively, was to be there, in the moment, without condition. Just be there . . . for whatever came next.

The continued aggressive care by ICU surgeons kept Angela alive through the long Thanksgiving weekend and the following week. I do not want to, nor can I, describe every medical procedure in detail. There were so many: the respirator, incisions for chest tubes, powerful antibiotics to fight multiple infections, further tests, needles, and more. I cannot remember all the tubes stuck into Angie's fragile body. Her lungs were being destroyed. Yet, she fought for life when everybody thought she could not survive. Because of that, Linda and I fought on along with her. When she was done, she would be done. We could not give up yet. We interpreted Angie's survival through the past weeks as her desire to live. No one else had a better answer.

During those critical days, we said thousands of prayers. The Anointing of the Sick sacrament was performed again. The hospital chaplain, Fr. Steve, was truly a compassionate friend and spiritual advisor. He gave us strength and love as Angela, somehow, survived the days of late November and early December.

J.D. told Linda and me that he was now going to take a leave from his job to devote his time to Angie for as long as she or Linda and I needed him, or until she was better. J.D. worked for his grandfather who owned a company that sponsored sports shows throughout the Midwest. His grandfather also loved Angela and supported J.D.'s decision, giving him complete latitude to be away from his job to be with her for as long as necessary. J.D.'s grandparents cared for Torrance while J.D. was at the hospital.

J.D. was with Angie eight to twelve hours each day. He arrived early each afternoon, often bringing the memory scrapbook Angie made for him, and he stayed late into the night. He spent hours with Angie, watching her fight for her life. He sat with Linda and me and other visiting friends in the waiting lounge hour after hour. He went to pick up our dinners on many nights. For a twenty-three-year-old man to be so devoted to his friend that he spent every day at Angie's bedside as the excruciating reality unfolded was amazing to Linda and me—J.D. was key to our survival during these weeks. The surroundings were so difficult, yet Linda and I were awed at his kindness and devotion. Angela was a hero, but so was her friend J.D.

Marcia Gallant adds…

On Thanksgiving 2002, Josh called to tell me the news about Angie. How could she be in a coma? I had only just talked with her online a couple of days before! At that point the doctors didn't think Angie would make it through the week, so I arranged to take my final exams early and flew back to Minnesota in December, hoping to see her before she passed. During that visit I spent most of my waking hours with Don, Linda, and J.D. in the waiting room.

One day I was alone with Angie in her hospital room, talking to her. I told her what I'd been up to, and that I'd just become engaged. I told her the next time I was supposed to see her was for my wedding, not in the hospital! As I stood next to her bed, I saw a tear roll from the corner of her eye, down her cheek. Seeing that teardrop made me feel that she knew I was with her, that I had come all that way to see her. A person in a coma may not be able to hear, let alone comprehend what is going on around them, but I felt in my heart that Angie knew I was there. I believe she knew how much her friends loved her.

Each day seemed to bring more grim news about Angie's condition. New strains of pseudomonas were identified in December; some were resistant to antibiotics. Angie's CO_2 levels remained precariously high. I met daily with doctors and tried to understand every step of the care and every decision being considered. On Friday, December 13, Angela was having a particularly tough day with CO_2 levels especially high. Her body was becoming acidic again. For the third time in three and a half weeks, doctors told Linda and me that Angela was likely in her final hours. We chose again to fight along with Angela. We'd give her every opportunity for life. The ICU doctors explored several options to bring her CO_2 levels down. Miraculously, they succeeded. Angela "stabilized" at a "very critical" level. These were the same words we had heard for weeks.

Weeks of living in Angie's hospital room and an ICU waiting lounge was taking a toll on our ability to sleep. Linda and I shared the available couches with other patients' family members. Occasionally we slept on the floor, on windowsills, or on whatever surface we could find. I awoke in the middle of each night and walked to Angie's room to check on her. I'd done the same routine so many times when she was small, struggling with a cold or infection. Now each night I walked down the empty hospital hallway to Angie's room. Usually only a nurse and a resident or intern were on duty. I put my hand on Angie's forehead and told her I loved her more than life itself. I said a prayer, then returned to my "bed of choice" for that night, and slept a couple more hours.

DREAM

I have been awakened from a dream
The cruel nature makes me ashamed

Life is so precious
As are the ones we love
But I am often blinded
By my own selfishness

Trivial, unimportant, self-absorbed
It seems only tragedy striking
Makes a difference and God
Hits closer and closer to home

Master of the universe — even mine
Planning on a timetable separate
Testing every single one of us
When we least expect it

We must remain strong and lean
On one another come what may
Seldom understanding but thanking
When all turns out as we hoped

Sometimes the answer is no
Though nobody wants to hear it
So we must pray again and again
Never turning away in confusion

I have been awakened by a dream
Now is the time to support each other

Brian J. Kuhl © 2002

Angela's cousin, Brian Kuhl, was a frequent visitor to the hospital.
He was the same age as Angie, and they had played together often as kids.

S O MANY FAMILY MEMBERS and friends supported us through our many weeks living in the ICU. Linda's family organized a group that came several times a week to help us pass the hours. They drove more than an hour each time. The same was true of my sister Joan and her husband, Bill. Joan earned a reputation on 4D for her delicious cooking, sharing food weekly with everyone present. Thanks to Joan's cooking, deliveries from area restaurants, and take-out meals from several of our favorite restaurants, we had sufficient breaks from hospital cafeteria food.

Grant and Kathi were at our side almost daily. They frequently brought their three children to visit Angie. Their twelve-year-old daughter was mature beyond her years. She came often even though she hadn't known Angie before then. She paid close attention to the tubes and contraptions in Angie's room. Her youthful chatter brought a welcome break to the emotional tension for us and for other families in 4D.

Dick and Jeanne Johnson, our friends for about sixteen years, rearranged their lives and schedules to be with us virtually every evening. They both were with us whenever we needed advice and support. Jeanne got to know everyone in the 4D lounge. She learned entire life stories after only a conversation or two. Dick stayed late each night, frequently until the morning. He knew when to be an advocate for Angela, a surrogate for me, or a confidante with sage advice and thoughtful counsel. We shared many hours, walking hospital corridors, discussing Angela, her care, and the gruesome circumstances. Dick and I often discussed the doctors' recommendation to let Angela go since her lungs had no chance of recovery.

Angela fought hard for life. We wanted to make the best decisions for her. The doctors assured us that she was not in pain nor aware of her condition. So, until we were certain a contrary decision was best for Angie, we had to choose life. A miracle recovery was always possible. Linda and I were so frightened by Angie's prognosis and the extent of the aggressive care she required hour by hour, keeping our minds clear was crucial so that we could make any life-and-death decisions without ambiguity.

Dick Johnson was the perfect person to provide us with clear thinking. He spent enough hours with Linda and me to fully understand the circumstances surrounding Angela's condition. He continued to encourage me to pursue life for as long as possible. He pointed out that when life is over, life is over—no matter what the afterlife brings. With the loss of my parents, my brother and many friends, I understood the finality that death brings. Dick supported us without reservation in this crucial decision to fight for Angie's life.

THE FIRST TWO WEEKS OF DECEMBER presented so many difficult circumstances and challenging decisions. I had never experienced such enormous stress. We had just endured a terrifying Thanksgiving and now Christmas was coming. Would we spend the holiday season in the hospital or at home—without Angela? By mid-December, Linda and I were prepared to live in the ICU forever if doing so was in Angela's best interests.

PART FOUR

THE
FAMILY
ROOM

A sign in the hallway outside the 4D waiting lounge read: Heroism consists of hanging on for one minute longer. Miracles occurred there frequently. Courageous lives ended there often as well. Some deaths were anticipated and some occurred unexpectedly. Some had family and friends surrounding them constantly and some appeared to be primarily or totally alone in their suffering. If a patient didn't exit 4D within days of surgery, one could assume they had encountered major, life-threatening complications.

By mid-December, Angela had held on for weeks. She had been totally sedated for more than a month, on a ventilator, with eleven chest tubes. She was our courageous hero long before then, but she now far exceeded any definition of courage established at 4D.

Linda and I exercised Angie's legs every day, spoke to her while we were with her, and tried to think of anything we could do to help her. The doctor ordered her regular hospital bed to be replaced with an air mattress bed designed to prevent pressure wounds for patients who could not move. Linda rubbed moisturizing lotion on Angie's skin and massaged her feet. Rehab folks came three times a week and told us things we could do to help keep Angie's muscles and tendons from becoming tight. I held her hands, stretched her fingers, and exercised her arms and legs at least twice every day.

Though Angela's stay was clearly unique in duration and extreme critical nature, we met many individuals and families in 4D who were facing their own medical crises or the crisis of a loved one. Family members spent their ongoing waiting time in the 4D lounge, reading, watching television or staring at the walls. Many reached out to support others and received support in return. Linda and I were blessed beyond measure with love and companionship from friends and family, and we developed relationships with some unforgettable people we encountered in 4D.

WE HAD ONLY BEEN IN THE ICU WORLD for about a week when we struck up a friendship with Bob and Lois from New Richmond, Wisconsin. Bob's brother, Leroy, experienced severe post-surgical complications. His condition was critical, and his body was slowly shutting down. Bob had a warm smile and kind eyes. Despite the loss facing him, he agonized quietly with Linda and me for the severity of our situation and the loss we were facing.

One afternoon I saw Bob and his wife sitting in the main lobby of the hospital. I stopped for a moment to talk with them. Tears welled up in Bob's eyes as he said he decided to withhold life support from his brother. Leroy was to die that afternoon. Bob could not watch. He and Lois were waiting in the lobby for confirmation of his brother's death. The stark reality of the whole awful environment overcame me. I held my emotions until I found a quiet place in the hospital to be alone. I returned later and was with Bob when he was given the news. I told him how sorry I felt. I could read in his eyes that he knew I would soon likely experience my own devastating loss. Bob had a compassionate heart. His was the first of many sad endings for families we met in the 4D lounge. Bob's family's loss brought home to Linda and me how painful a decision to end life support for Angela would be.

Another family to enter this unique existence had arrived the day after Thanksgiving. Earlier that day, Darvin, a farmer from the small town of Harvey, North Dakota, had received word that his wife, Sandra, had suffered a heart attack. She had been treated briefly in North Dakota, but was soon airlifted to University Hospital for the implantation of a heart pump, to be followed by a heart transplant. Darvin had driven all day to Minneapolis, a city with which he was entirely unfamiliar. He had been directed to the wrong hospital, and then had negotiated rush-hour traffic to reach the right one.

By the time Darvin arrived, he was clearly confused and concerned. The first person he met as he came off the fourth floor elevator was our friend, Jeanne Johnson—the perfect person for him to encounter. Jeanne immediately recognized Darvin as a man in despair and in need of a "guide" to find the answers to his many questions about his wife's condition. Soon, we were friends with Darvin. We spent our days together, over many long weeks. He was a fine man with a true and big heart. His wife was occasionally moved from the ICU to a room, but she continued to have serious, life-threatening complications during her recovery that brought her back to the ICU. On many days we stood at Darvin's side, praying for a "miracle" outcome for Sandra. And Darvin prayed for us and supported us in Angela's jeopardy.

Every evening, Linda and I, along with any visiting family and friends, gathered in the 4D lounge or the hospital cafeteria for dinner. We always asked Darvin to join us; our invitations were accepted with his gentle, thankful smile. Dick Johnson, J.D., Darvin, Linda, and I were together almost every night.

CHRISTMAS WAS COMING SOON to 4D. Linda and I had lived there now for more than a month. While the struggle for Angie's life had its ebbs and flows, Angie was never removed from a "gravely critical" or "hour-to-hour" status. Her miraculous fight for life was astonishing, and physically and emotionally exhausting for Linda and me and our supportive family and friends. I often thought about the stress on each of us involved in this horrible experience. But, whatever had to be endured to be at Angela's side was nothing compared to what she was enduring and would likely have to encounter ahead. The whole scene was breaking our hearts, but Linda and I were right where we wanted to be—with our beloved Angie. Nothing else mattered.

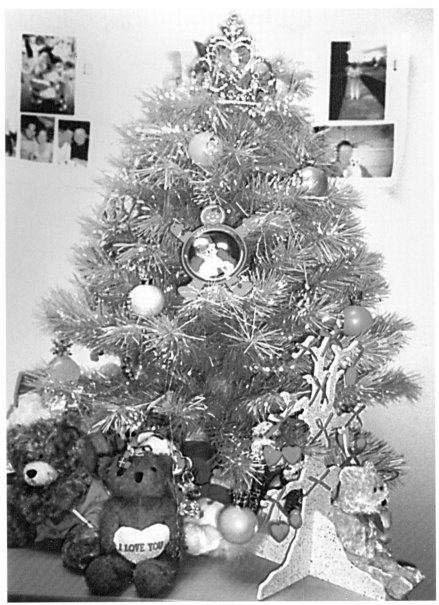

Linda decorated a Christmas tree that she placed beside Angie's hospital bed.

THE DAY BEFORE CHRISTMAS, we were informed that Dr. Eddy was on vacation during the holidays and Dr. George would temporarily take over Angela's care. Dr. Eddy had been Angie's primary pulmonologist for about six years since Dr. Warren Warwick turned seventy years old and began limiting his practice. Dr. Eddy was familiar with Angie, and we had been meeting with him several times a week. We held out hope that he and the surgical ICU team could still pull off a miracle. With Dr. Eddy gone, we relied primarily on the ICU team, and our confidence in the ICU team never waned.

As with every other day, Linda and I spent Christmas Eve at the hospital. Angela loved Christmas so much. She always inspired Linda and me to be fully "in the spirit" of the holiday, even when we were tired of the activities, crowds, and shopping. I was so sad that Angie lay unconscious on her favorite holiday. Linda and I decided to go to a Christmas Eve Mass at 4:00 P.M. in the chapel on the eighth floor of the hospital.

The chapel was quiet. Candles were burning and a table served as an altar. About a dozen or so patients and family members were present, including Margaret, a friend from 4D, and one of her daughters. Father Steve performed the Mass by candlelight. He had become a close friend as he prayed with Linda and me almost daily.

Father Steve dedicated this Christmas Eve Mass to Angela and told her story with loving and heartfelt emotion. The poignancy of his message of love and God's will kept us in tears. Most of those present already knew about Angela. Fr. Steve described an intelligent, beautiful, twenty-one-year-old girl laying in a bed four floors below, breathing for the fifth week on a ventilator, in a medicated coma, and with eleven chest tubes—a disturbing image. The eyes of all those present were soon trained on us. Everyone wept with us, hearing about Angela's struggle for life. Linda and I cried throughout the beautiful Mass. We tried to sing the chosen carols, but we could not get through them. We were touched with gratitude for the outpouring of love around us that night.

Margaret and her daughter made frequent eye contact with us in our sorrow. She and her children and their spouses had entered the Family Room shortly before Christmas. The family owned a dairy farm in Marshfield, Wisconsin. Margaret's husband had received a mechanical heart pump. Just like Darvin's wife, Margaret's husband would eventually need a heart transplant. We had shared many days full of conversation and friendly support. Our relationship with Margaret's family deepened further during the Christmas Eve service. Margaret and others greeted us warmly when the Mass finished.

When Linda and I returned to 4D after the Mass, Joan and Bill were waiting for us. We were discussing going to the cafeteria for dinner when a nurse came to the lounge. With a grave look on her face she told us Angela was "having problems." She was bleeding up through her breathing tube, which meant hemorrhaging in her lungs. We rushed to her room to find several nurses surrounding her bed, working feverishly. Two nurses had blood saturating the front of their exam gowns. We were asked to remain outside the door. I caught a glimpse of a resident squeezing a manual ventilator and the clinicians appeared to be suctioning like crazy.

One of the ICU doctors came out to tell Linda and me, again, that Angie was not likely to live through the night. This night was Christmas Eve. Would our daughter die on Christmas Eve? Angela loved Christmas. We began calls to family and friends to tell them of her grave status.

An emergency call went out to the on-call pulmonologist. But, by mistake, the pediatric pulmonologist on call was summoned—that was Warren Warwick. Dr. Warwick had not been involved in Angela's care for many years, but he had seen Angela during her October 2002 hospitalization, just two months earlier. The mistaken request for Dr. Warwick to come to the hospital was quickly cancelled, but Dr. Warwick, upon learning that Angela was the patient in distress, came to the hospital anyway.

As Joan, Bill, Linda, and I waited anxiously, Dr. Warwick walked into the 4D lounge. With him was one of his daughters. He was dressed in a tuxedo. Formal dress was part of his family's Christmas Eve tradition. We were touched that he chose to see Angie and be with Linda and me during this time of crisis, especially knowing he'd left his family on an important holiday. We sat in the 4D lounge, which was practically empty that night. We cried together and talked about Dr. Warwick's almost fifty years of fighting cystic fibrosis and our twenty-one-plus years of fighting the disease. We talked about how much Angie had been through. She had already endured five weeks on a ventilator and now had eleven chest tubes. Dr. Warwick stayed with us until after 9:00 P.M. Before he left, I asked him, "How will we know when enough is enough?"

He answered, "With CF, you never give up—you must fight until the end with this disease, for there is no other way to eventually succeed."

Dr. Warwick's advice supported what Linda and I had always believed throughout our lives with Angie. A truth for every person who battles against cystic fibrosis is that it is a daily fight with no rest.

I spoke to Linda's mother by phone that night. When I told her that Angela was not expected to survive the night, Bernelda's deep Catholic faith was evident as she tried to comfort us, saying, "What a glorious day—Christmas—for Angie to go to Heaven!"

Josh and others came to the hospital. Dick and Jeanne joined us around midnight for our nightlong vigil. Sometime during the night, the bleeding in Angela's lungs stopped. Christmas morning arrived, and Angela was still alive.

I knew in my heart that as bad as the past weeks had been, the situation was likely to become worse for Angie. Although I continued to pray for a miracle and I was willing to stay at 4D and fight for Angie until my own death, I was quite conscious of the impending predicament awaiting Linda and me. This distorted and horrible Christmas was likely our last with Angie on Earth.

Linda's family and my business partner, Grant, and his family shared Christmas day with us. Despite moments of joy and laughter, Linda's and my thoughts remained in the nearby room where Angie lay with the rhythmic beat of the respirator and the constant bubbling sound of the water tanks attached to each of eleven chest tubes. The bubbles rising in the water was the air leaking from Angie's lungs. To share Christmas at 4D with our loved ones and the families of other patients, most of whom we would not see again, seemed oddly normal.

We had conversations through the day with doctors about the medical crisis the previous evening. They expressed concern about what the bleeding in the ventilator tube indicated regarding tissue breakdown in Angela's lungs. We were again asked how much more we were prepared to do while awaiting a miracle for Angie. So many people were there for Angela and us. Christmas was not the day to make the decision to quit; we told the doctors we wanted to fight on.

Two of the physicians on the ICU team talked to us about the possibility of doing a tracheotomy on Angela, placing the ventilator breathing tube through her trachea. In addition, they could place a feeding tube directly into her stomach. The procedures, if we approved, could be done the next day in the ICU since there was too much risk in transferring her to an operating room. The tubes in Angela's mouth and nose would be gone, but there was also a one-in-five chance that Angela would not survive the two procedures. After a brief discussion, we decided to go forward. Linda and I had complete confidence in the skills of the ICU surgeons. So the procedures were scheduled for December 26 at 10:30 A.M. Linda and I found couches in another lounge on the fourth floor. Sleeping was difficult Christmas night, knowing that tomorrow would be another day of crisis and risk.

In the morning we were at Angie's side early, remembering the one-in-five odds. Once again, friends and family were at our side. Bill and Joan returned, as did Dick Johnson, Grant, Josh, and J.D. Grant's wife, Kathi, sent trays of appetizers for everyone. Linda and I were humbled once again by our network of loving supporters.

As the procedure began, Linda and I held hands. Our hearts and minds were in Angie's room with her. Participating in the idle conversation everyone tried to provide was hard. I could only imagine a doctor coming to tell us Angie had not survived the surgery.

An hour passed and then an hour and a half. More than once we walked by Angela's room and peeked through a small opening in the curtain. All we could see was the ICU doctor behind Angela operating a manual ventilator.

Finally, nearly two hours later, the two doctors came to the waiting lounge and told us everything had gone well. Angie had done well. Linda and I cried in relief and went to see her. While no significant change had occurred in her medical condition, the visual image of our daughter without a feeding tube in her nose or a breathing tube in her mouth was especially comforting.

Her beautiful face looked perfect and peaceful. Linda and I could not hold in our emotions. The ordeal was still horrible but, as least now, we could see and touch and stroke Angie's face unobstructed. We were now able to hold her face and kiss her freely. Dozens of times each day I held my open hand over her entire forehead and gently stroked her perfect little nose. When alone with her, I caressed her face while praying for her and telling her how much I loved her.

Linda was comforted and excited to see Angie looking so much more at peace. We presumed Angela's comfort was improved but we really had no idea how she was feeling. To our surprise, within days, her lung function and blood test results improved. She still remained in the status of "extremely critical" with no realistic hope of survival, but for the first time since Thanksgiving morning, she was not labeled "hour to hour." The ICU staff now referred to her condition as "shift to shift"—an "inside ICU" definition. Our hope for a miracle had, at least, a breath of chance.

Over the next week, Angie's lung function stabilized. Her lungs were still ravaged and she remained critical, but she was absorbing sufficient oxygen and releasing enough carbon dioxide, and her vital organs were performing well. Her body and her soul were surviving heroically.

On December 30, Dr. George wanted to speak with Linda and me. He proposed that Angela's only chance for survival was a lobar transplant but such a transplant could be contemplated only if her condition continued to improve… and if Angie awoke. Both were big ifs. Two healthy donors were needed to each donate one lobe of their lungs. In the transplant procedure, the recipient's natural lungs are removed and replaced by a single donor lobe on each side. When the transplant is completed, the patient is given high doses of anti-rejection drugs that also suppress the immune system and lessen the patient's ability to fight infection. While a ventilator performs the temporary breathing, the lungs are more vulnerable to infection as the lungs and airways are exposed to outside bacteria. If infection can be avoided, eventually the new lungs expand to fill the chest cavity to function at seventy percent or more of normal. Most importantly, the new lungs would be free of CF. Lobar lung transplants were a relatively new procedure. At University Hospital, only a handful had been attempted, with minimal success. Such a transplant was a long shot—and our last hope.

For two people who had been praying for a miracle for about fifty days, these were words that lifted Linda's and my spirits. I immediately called upon friends to do as much research as possible on lobar transplants.

AT ABOUT 6:00 P.M. on New Year's Eve, alarms sounded on 4D, indicating a patient needed to be resuscitated. Being a holiday, the staff was not at full capacity. We tried to stay out of the way during such frantic times, but we soon learned that Margaret's husband had suffered cardiac arrest and passed away. Hearing this, Linda looked for Margaret. We had noticed earlier in the evening that she was alone at the hospital without any of her children. Now her children would not arrive from Marshfield for two hours. Linda and I found her mourning alone in a small conference room. Her grief and sorrow were evident as she sat with her head down.

Linda and I stayed with Margaret until her family arrived. I was so moved, seeing this loving family in grief. Yet even in their time of sadness they consoled us, knowing our stay in 4D was not over. With each family's departure, new families also joined us in the "Family Room."

ONCE I HAD BEGUN passing the word that Angela might be a candidate for a lobar lung transplant, potential donors came forward. Josh immediately offered. Another family friend had her blood tested to see if her type was compatible, and Linda was also a possible donor. We were aware that Angela's condition had to improve first, but we wanted to be ready if and when that happened. We informed Dr. George of our success in finding willing donors. Now that we had blood-type matches, we were ready for the next series of compatibility tests required by the transplant clinic.

But Dr. George now downplayed the possibility of a lobar transplant for Angela. Her condition was far from transplant acceptable. He was not convinced she would ever be well enough. We were confused by his changed tone. Angela's condition was not good, but his suggestion about the possibility of a lobar lung transplant had given us hope that she might improve over the coming days or weeks, and if she did, we could still pursue this option. We were quietly angry that this doctor had raised our hopes and those of family and friends if a transplant was a completely unrealistic option.

As our last hope began to dissolve in early January, the inevitable became more obvious. Our hopes were fading as Angie's condition failed to improve any further in the coming days. We had much emotional and mental preparation to process before we could say goodbye to our beloved Angela.

ON JANUARY 10, 2003, a young woman from South Dakota entered the hospital to receive a lobar lung transplant. Lisa, who was twenty-seven years old, also had cystic fibrosis. Her lungs were failing and a transplant was her only option. Two young, healthy men, Lisa's husband and a co-worker, were donating lobes for her. Her chances sounded good. If her transplant succeeded, her lungs would be free of cystic fibrosis.

The optimism surrounding Lisa and her family was both encouraging and bittersweet for us. Our hopes were raised by her story, though she was not in critical condition like Angie. Lisa was alert, mobile, and not on a ventilator. Would she have a chance at a lifesaving transplant, but not Angela? We still prayed and hoped for Angie to improve sufficiently to have her own opportunity for a lifesaving transplant. Though peculiar to pray for our child to undergo a high-risk, painful surgery and recovery, the faint possibility was all we had.

On the day of Lisa's surgery, her family filled the 4D lounge. They were concerned yet optimistic. They were aware of Angela's condition and our desperate hopes, making them acutely sensitive to the circumstances from our perspective: we sincerely wanted Lisa's surgery to be successful and to be followed by a successful transplant for Angela. Our two families shared our "war" stories about fighting CF, as well as our hopes for the future.

Lisa's transplant surgery was a success and she came back to 4D on a ventilator. Lisa's family hoped her new lobes would take over quickly and the ventilator could be removed. They also were aware that CF patients on ventilators were at risk. I cringed to think that Angela had been on a ventilator for almost two months by now.

The Family Room

Welcome to your new address
Leave life as you knew it at the door
Your stay will be indefinite
In room "D" on the 4th Floor
The waiting room? The worry room
Is what they should call this space
Sitting still and pacing slow
Strangers gather seeking grace
The waiting room, the worry room
Impatience feeds the fear
Of some news to come, prognosis waits
Son's fate drawing near
First words are spoken casually
Hours pass, time creeps by slow
The mood is dark with tension
All heads are hanging low
The worry room walls are built of pain
That surrounds the fragile heart
Of each and every loved one
Playing their supportive part
A discontent air fills the room
At times it's hard to breathe
You shift your weight and pace about
But your heart won't let you leave
Doubts and questions rule your head
Your spirit lacks control
A day evolves into a week
Time brutally takes its toll
You expect the walls to smother you
Before uncertainty finds an end
But conversation takes a turn

As strangers become friends
With them comes increasing hope
You sense you're not alone
Hidden deep within the walls
Was family yet unknown
Reaching out to pull you in
Shared values are the glue
To the connection that we felt
When we first encountered you
The vulnerability in your eyes
The intimate nature of your strength
Your vow to beat this circumstance
To be here at any length
A similar vow is made by us
You have somewhere to lean
While days turn into weeks
And futures remain unseen
The waiting room? The family room
Is what they should call this space
Son's fate brings us together
We are blessed by your grace
Life as you knew it has been changed
As you exit the 4th Floor
We're here for you indefinitely
You are welcome always at our door
The wrong place at the right time
A space once filled with gloom
Open heart and renewed spirit
Built a family room

Amanda Roy © 2003

A couple of days after Lisa's transplant surgery, word spread through the floor that she had contracted an infection in her new lungs. The family was meeting with doctors. Deep concern pervaded the 4D lounge area. We watched as Lisa's family gathered together in her room. Less than a week after her surgery Lisa passed away from the infection that overwhelmed her new lungs. Her family did not return to the Family Room. Our last hope for a successful outcome for Angela faded with their silent departure.

IN THE MIDST OF OUR FEAR and grief about Angie's poor prognosis, another family crossed paths with us in the 4D lounge, "The Family Room." Though many stories intersected in the 4D lounge, none was more meaningful for me than knowing the family of Arthur Roy.

The first member of the Roy family I met was Amanda, a vivacious, sweet, beautiful and soulful young woman. She had accompanied her family to University Hospital shortly after New Year's Day from Casper, Wyoming, to support her thirty-three-year-old brother, Travis, who was to undergo an experimental surgery to slow the progress of an aggressive brain tumor. Travis's family also included his father, Arthur, his mother, brother, wife, and two children. They were a family united in a fight to save the life of their much-loved Travis.

During Travis's two-week hospital stay, Amanda connected easily with everyone around her. We spent many hours sharing stories that brought us together. From the time

Amanda and her family learned about Angela's situation, I sensed her story strongly affected Travis's father, Arthur. But, with so much tension and worry in 4D, I did not think much more about his unspoken reaction. Of course, Arthur was frightened about the future for his son, Travis, and Linda and I feared for Angela. Ours was a relationship bond that was common among long-term residents of 4D.

One night in the 4D lounge, Amanda shared with me her father's history with cystic fibrosis. Arthur had grown up in a family that knew CF too well. Three of his six siblings had died of CF, one at a year old, another at nineteen, and his brother at age thirty-eight. Amanda shared with me that being confronted with the reality of Angela's future, Arthur was reliving horrifying memories from his own past.

While Arthur and I were close to the same age, he reminded me of my father. Arthur was handsome, strong, an agricultural product salesman, and not one to share his deepest feelings with strangers. He and I spoke only a few times during Travis's stay, for neither of us were good at looking into the eyes of another man and seeing fear and pain. We both sensed the helplessness and sadness of the other.

When Travis was ready to return to Wyoming, his prognosis was uncertain. Only time would tell whether the surgery had slowed the course of his brain tumor. On the day the Roys left, Arthur came to me as I stood in the hallway outside Angela's room. He presented me with the book *Celebrate through Heartsongs* by poet Mattie Stepanek. The author suffered from severe muscular dystrophy [and died in 2004 at the age of thirteen]. Inside the cover Arthur wrote the following message:

"65 ROSES"

Known by families of children with CF, the term "65 roses" was first said by the young son of a volunteer for the Cystic Fibrosis Foundation in 1965. All three young sons of Mary Weiss had CF. When she asked her four-year-old what he thought his mother was working for, he had answered, "65 Roses." His pronunciation became widely used by children to describe the disease, and 65 Roses® became a registered trademark of the Cystic Fibrosis Foundation, which thereafter adopted the rose as its symbol.

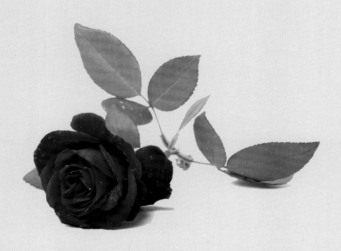

To our 'Kindred Spirits,' the Warners, from the Roy Family,

We wish you love, understanding, and deep feelings of compassion as you continue your struggle. Please know you are in our thoughts and prayers each day and that each of many contributions I will make in the future to the Cystic Fibrosis Foundation will be made with a special prayer from a family and to a family only too familiar with the true meaning of 65 Roses.

Your Kindred Spirits,

The Roy Family

Once the Roys returned to Wyoming, Amanda called the 4D lounge every few days to inquire about Angela, Linda and me.

THE GIFT

In our hearts and our minds, Linda and I always knew the most likely outcome for Angie, but knowing did not stop us from fighting on, aggressively pursuing every medical possibility, and continuously praying for a miracle. By January 16, with our hopes and dreams for a lobar transplant rapidly fading, Linda and I had one final meeting with yet another pulmonologist. Angela had to improve further before a major transplant surgery could be considered. Though we had no reason to believe this would happen, Linda and I wanted to make sure we had discussed every option before giving up on the possibility of a miracle.

Dr. Marshall Hertz was an expert in lung transplantation and a professor of medicine at the University of Minnesota. He was a friend of Dick and Jeanne Johnson, and while not directly involved with Angela's care, he had taken an interest at the request of Dick and Jeanne. We met with him in a small office on the fourth floor. He quickly gained our trust as he demonstrated sincere compassion for Angie and for Linda and me, speaking to us directly, giving us the benefit of his knowledge and experience.

Dr. Hertz explained that medical ethics ruled out the idea of taking lung lobes from healthy people and giving them to someone who would likely not survive. Angie's chances were slim based on her current condition. He confirmed that for her to be able to undergo a transplant attempt, she not only had to regain consciousness but also be able to participate in some physical therapy preparation.

By the end of our discussion with Dr. Hertz, we knew what we had to do. In recent weeks, some of the chest tubes had been removed. Now there were only four. The removal of each tube was a small victory that gave us a shred of hope, causing us, in a final act of desperation, to try to reduce Angie's sedation and wake her up.

This would be physically hard on Angela, and medically difficult after so many weeks. Waking her had to be done slowly, with close monitoring of her progress. The ICU doctors predicted that the process might take up to a week to wean her gradually from the amount of sedation she had been on. Oh, how I wanted to see those beautiful, alert eyes again, one more time. But another part of me did not want to see the fear and pain that would surely be in her eyes as well.

Linda and I continued to maintain our belief that Angie loved life and would want to live under almost any circumstances. As long as her body was fighting for life, we would fight with her and for her. We felt Angie would somehow "tell" us when the fight was over. So, the wake up attempt began.

On the second or third day into the attempt, Angie's head began to shift and jolt side to side, and twice her eyes opened reflexively. Her blood pressure began to rise, indicating her increasing stress level. She began trying to override the ventilator with her own breathing. The nurses told us these were merely reflexive actions but they did indicate that a complete awakening would be difficult, dangerous, and very stressful for Angie.

After only three days we could see that waking Angie to pursue the remote chance that she would survive a very risky lobar transplant was not what Linda or I could do to our daughter. With the support of her doctors, the decision was made to stop trying to wake her and to let her rest peacefully, for now. After a week or two of wishful expectation, our hopes and options were ending as the prospects for a lobar transplant finally evaporated.

SINCE WAKING ANGIE WAS NOT POSSIBLE, the end was now only a matter of time and circumstance. Almost a week passed before Linda and I had the conversation about where to go from there. I suggested to Linda that the "final great gift of love" we could give Angie might be to control the timing, conditions, and circumstances of her final moments before going to Heaven. The other option was to continue to pray for a miracle while taking the risk that her end would come traumatically at a moment when Linda and/or I were not there. We had continually feared that would happen. Not being with Angie at the end was an unacceptable option. We wanted to be with her and hold her in her final moments. Her body could not hold out forever with her damaged lungs. The doctors told us again: there was no realistic chance of her survival.

Linda met privately with a trusted ICU physician on February 1 in the afternoon. The doctor gave Linda assurances that the "gift" we were considering was the right choice for Angie. I had a similar meeting with the head of the ICU surgical team. The decision was made to give our little girl, the greatest love of our lives, the "gift" of a peaceful final journey to that "incomprehensible and unimaginable" Heaven. Linda and I would have given anything to trade places with Angie. We tentatively chose February 6, 2003, as the day. We reserved the right to change our minds.

Within a day or so of making the most horrific decision a parent can be asked to make, we received a small amount of consolation that our decision was the only one available to us. Angela's beautiful and fragile body finally began to give out. She had truly been a gallant and heroic warrior against CF her entire life, particularly the past eighty-one days. We were now told that her kidneys and digestive tract were beginning to fail. In some way the three of us had decided together that now was the time for our child to go to Heaven. Angie was showing us the way.

On Monday, February 3, we let our family and a few friends know of the timing. J.D. notified some of Angela's friends. We met with the director of the funeral home we had chosen weeks earlier when doctors first told us Angie had only hours to live. On Tuesday we spent the afternoon at a casket manufacturer, selecting just the right "treasure chest." We called the casket a treasure chest after our priest told us the story of the little boy who, attending a funeral for another child, asked his mother about the casket.

His mother said the box was a treasure chest with contents of great value. When the boy asked when they could open the treasure chest, his mother said, "Only Jesus gets to open it."

We continued to ask questions as each day passed. We talked to our spiritual advisors, our family and friends, as well as the doctors involved in Angie's care.

After the last eighty-plus days of horror and hope, those two or three final days were spent in shock, walking in a surreal stupor, interrupted by a good cry every few hours. We survived those days because of our love for Angela and the love and support of our family and friends. Dick Johnson and J.D. made themselves available again at any time during the day or night to be with Angela if Linda and I had to leave the hospital to carry out some of the difficult planning tasks together.

Even with emotional and mental preparation, there was no way to be ready for the last day. So many lives were about to change forever on that day—the day Angela was to begin her eternal journey, without us.

By 5:00 P.M. on Wednesday, February 5, 2003, Linda and I confirmed the final decision: tomorrow we would allow our daughter, Angela, to be released from her earthly pain and suffering. After eighty-six days in the 4D Intensive Care Unit of the University of Minnesota Medical Center, we knew which nurse we wanted present for such an excruciating event and which doctor we wanted to supervise those final moments so they would be as painless and controlled for Angie as possible. Based on those factors and others, Linda and I chose 3:00 P.M. on February 6, 2003. The countdown of hours, and eventually minutes, began.

Cystic fibrosis had won this war. As difficult as the next twenty or so hours would be, we had no other choice but to love Angie beyond belief, hold her and cherish her, and pray for God to rush her to the glories of Heaven.

Wednesday night was the longest night of our lives. Dick and Jeanne Johnson were there to stay with us through the night. They had altered and devoted their lives for months to see us through our darkest hours. Grant and Kathi joined our all-night vigil.

We spent the evening talking, calling family and friends who might wish to be present the next day, and lying in bed alongside Angela, holding her. With some of her aggressive respiratory therapies halted, we were able to freely hold her in our arms for the first time in months. She seemed so fragile, and I wondered if she could sense our presence on some level after eleven weeks of heavy sedation and having been on ventilator life support for almost three months. While we hoped she could feel our love and presence, we did not want her to feel the pain that was likely, or to be terrified about what the next day would bring. Linda and I could have gone on loving and holding Angie forever, whispering comforting and loving words in her ears.

The hours ticked by much too fast as we approached the appointed time. We both wanted to stay with Angela all evening and all night. In the morning we would have to share her with friends and family who also wanted to be with her before she left us. Our love affair with this beautiful young lady had begun almost twenty-two years earlier and would not ever end. But, the fact that our earthly path with her was about to end was unimaginable and indescribably painful for Linda and me. Our hearts were broken beyond repair.

After dreamlike, or more accurately, nightmarish, hours of lying in Angie's bed with her or roaming the hospital corridors and waiting lounge, morning finally arrived. The sun rose. This was the day our Angela would die. Those words went through my mind, but they seemed surreal. While those around us spoke of the scope and depth of our loss, our focus had always been on Angela throughout her life and remained so even at this terrible time. The loss to *her* haunted me. *She* was the one who would not experience the joy of this life any longer. *She* would not have the opportunity to marry or have children. *She* would no longer share good times with her friends, meet new friends, travel again to places she loved or play with her Maltese puppy, Torrance. *She* would not feel our hugs and kisses here on earth or those of her family and friends who also loved her so much. *She* would no longer walk on the beach.

Also gone was Angie's exhaustive daily regimen that was necessary to fight cystic fibrosis—the bronchial drainage therapies, the antibiotics and other pills, the occasional hospital stays, and the fight for each breath. Without future genetic therapy or a lung transplant, Angie's fight and survival would have required ever more strength and courage. Despite my desire to find something positive in our dear Angie leaving us, those thoughts were mere rationalizations. I wanted to make a horrible, tragic, sickening day a little less so. The rationalizations did not work. The pain filled my body, my mind, and my soul. Passing "The Family Room" I read again the message on the outside wall: *Heroism consists of hanging on for one more minute.*

Linda and I often agreed that Angie was a better, stronger, and more courageous person than either of us. She had been our hero her entire life. Though I suspect every CF parent rightly believes that their child's fight against the disease is heroic, I was always amazed by the quiet discipline Angie displayed, her lack of self-pity, her love and devotion to her flawed parents, and her genuine and lasting friendships. Her many achievements academically and athletically—despite cystic fibrosis—were secondary to her essence, which was her love and caring for others and her tireless commitment to fighting CF. Now she was losing the battle she fought so hard to win.

Family and friends began to arrive about 9:00 A.M. Dick and Jeanne and Grant and Kathi had gone to their homes for a brief rest, but others soon arrived. My sister Joan and her husband Bill arrived first. Soon after, J.D. arrived.

By 10:00 A.M. members of Linda's family began to arrive: Linda's mom and dad and Sister Dorothy, Linda's sister Judi and her daughters, Tracy and Terry, and Linda's younger brother Ron and his wife, Shannon, along with their children, Brian and Susan. All these people had gathered to say goodbye to Angela.

More and more friends arrived as the hours passed: J.D.'s mother, Holly, and his sister, Michelle, and many of Angela's friends, including Andrea, Lynn, and Dan. J.D. had kept them all informed of Angela's condition between their own visits. Soon twenty to thirty friends and family members were moving between Angie's room and the 4D lounge Family Room. Tension was felt everywhere.

In the late morning, J.D. left to bring Angie's cherished little dog, Torrance, to the hospital for a last goodbye. My breath caught in my throat as I recalled what Angie had said when she first brought Torrance home, a little more than a year before. In discussing the short life expectancy of dogs, Angie had commented that she would likely outlive her beloved Torrance.

J.D. returned with Torrance. The puppy was so elated to see Angela; he could not stop licking her motionless face. I hoped Angela could feel Torrance's presence on some subconscious level. J.D. took Torrance back home about 2:00 P.M. so he could return to the hospital for Angie's final moments.

Dick and Jeanne returned after resting, then Grant and Kathi, soon followed by Josh. Even family members of other ICU patients began migrating to our lounge. So many of them had become our friends through our long stay in 4D. Our Family Room friend Darvin gave us kind words and loving embraces during Angela's final hours. I was aware that everyone present had thought or known for weeks that this day was inevitable. Linda and I had fought this battle, which had defined so much of our lives for so long, with all the strength that we, and Angela, had. Today the fight was ending.

The time came to meet with the ICU physician, who would supervise the final moments, and with the physician head of the ICU. Both of these doctors had become our friends. They had shown compassion, knowledge, and deep understanding. Together they described the steps that would follow and what we should expect. They would increase the level of Angela's sedation to be certain there would be no chance of consciousness and to eliminate the possibility of anxiety. Oxygen levels provided by the ventilator would be reduced to room level. Angela's lungs had been so destroyed that room-level oxygen was "insufficient for life." The doctors estimated "it would be all over" in ten to twenty minutes once begun.

I was sickened to hear the process described again. The steps involved sounded so matter-of-fact, but the words were like explosions going off in my head. This just could not be happening—but it was! I thanked the doctors for their gentle souls and heroic efforts throughout Angie's ICU stay and for helping us navigate these final hours. Despite our concerns about some of the care Angela received prior to the abdominal surgery, the doctors in ICU had been magnificent.

About 2:45 P.M. our priest from Pax Christi Catholic Church, Father Tim Power, arrived along with Father Steve La Canne, the hospital priest. Fr. Tim and several representatives of Pax Christi had visited us and prayed with us often during Angela's hospitalization, and Fr. Tim had performed the Anointing of the Sick for Angela several times during her months of struggle. He had provided great counsel during the last days of decisions.

Fr. Steve's frequent hugs, prayers, and his friendship were great blessings to Linda and me. We felt comforted whenever he was present. Fr. Steve had become personally involved in the loss we were experiencing and the tragedy that was happening to Angela. His eyes showed his private pain, yet his words remained those of comfort and strength.

So, surrounding Angie at 3:00 P.M. were more than two dozen family members and friends, the ICU doctor, Angela's nurse, both priests and, in the far corner of the room, Dr. Warren Warwick. Linda lay down beside Angela and held her. I stood on the other side of the bed and held Angie's hand tightly. I put my head down on her shoulder with my mouth near her ear. When the time came I squeezed her hand and told her in whatever words came to me that I loved her beyond imagination and that I looked forward to reuniting with her soon for eternity.

At 3:15 P.M., Fr. Tim and Fr. Steve began a series of scripture readings and prayers. I remember the Lord's Prayer and the twenty-third Psalm. The Rosary was prayed with family and friends participating, even some of the non-Catholics. The priests performed the "Chant of the Saints." The lights were dimmed and soft music played in the background from a recording J.D. had made. Angela was given her final Last Rites. Two priests prayed for her soul and for all present who were living through unbearable grief and pain. Angie was in the arms of her adoring parents and loving family and friends. The scene was both beautiful and heartbreaking as her precious soul was about to take flight.

At 3:45 P.M., the doctor administered the additional sedatives and turned down the oxygen of the ventilator. Linda and I held Angie tight; I spoke to her continuously. I felt Grant's strong hands rubbing my back. Linda laid her head on Angie's chest to listen to her heart. Tears were flowing everywhere. I squeezed Angela's hand so hard I unknowingly caused bruising. I was so angry, frightened, and excruciatingly sad. In a few short minutes, it was over. I lifted my head from her ear and said to Linda, "Honey, she's gone."

This was the worst moment of the worst day of our lives. Our little girl was dead. I cannot adequately describe the pain and sadness. Angela was gone. How does anyone survive such a loss? We were going to find out.

LIFE

Life is not fair
I was reminded once again last evening

How one is chosen
And another passed over
Haunts me and others
When looking back on our gifts

Not only am I indebted
Bound through invisible ties
I must live to the fullest
These talents, moments, and opportunities

Guilt crouches in waiting
To prey on my damaged heart
Though I should not fear
For an omnipotent hand guides me

She has given so much to the world
Taken at a moment for a reason
One that continues to escape everyone
And tears seem to be the only comfort offered

I heard I must not give up hope
Follow the brave heroine's footsteps
Courageously face the words
I am afraid — yes we are too

Life is not fair
Close your eyes and let her lead

Brian J. Kuhl 2003

In those hours after Angie died, Darvin was so genuine and comforting. He came into the room, put his big calloused hands on our shoulders, and expressed his sorrow. Tears ran down his face. We hugged one another and expressed our love for each other. Ours was a closeness born out of crisis, that grew during shared horror, and became forever cemented by the most painful experiences one can face in life: the death of a child for Linda and me, and the possible death of a spouse for a man so devoted to his wife. For weeks we had shared our days together in the Family Room. Darvin and his wife, Sandra, left an indelible impression on our hearts.

Linda and I said goodbye to our faithful friends for the night and drove home, both of us crying most of the way. We had planned Angie's funeral and reception for Monday. There was still much to do. But, first, we needed to get through the night.

QUIETLY UNDER THE SURFACE

Arriving home Thursday evening felt so strange, knowing I would be staying for the night. I had slept in the ICU every night since before Thanksgiving 2002, and now it was February 6, 2003. My own bed was foreign but a welcome sight. How comforting to finally share the bed with Linda and hold her in my arms. But my mind focused on the empty bedroom down the hall. We needed to live through the first night.

Linda and I had driven home from the hospital in silence after Angie died. We unloaded the car full of our temporary living supplies, Angie's things and the gifts and mementos from loved ones. We headed to bed for the first of countless nights of tears, sleeplessness, nightmares, flashbacks, and physical illness. Thus began life with a broken heart.

THE DAYS THAT FOLLOWED were mostly a blur. Linda and I walked in the equivalent of a deep, dark fog. We went through the motions of planning the funeral and interment. Every decision was excruciating. This was so much different than a year earlier, when I had lost my mother. Picking out the last clothes our beautiful young daughter would wear was an unspeakable task.

I rotated from the cold accomplishment of duties necessary for arranging Angie's mass to spending hours in front of the television without knowing what I was watching. I stared at blank walls, cried in anguish, even wished for my own death. I could not imagine continuing to live with so much pain. I wanted to be wherever Angie was, so she would not be alone.

KNOWING FOR WEEKS that these days were likely, some advance planning had been done. We had already chosen a beautiful mausoleum and chapel that would be Angie's final resting place and one day, our own. Just before Christmas I had taken an afternoon away from the hospital to find an above-ground mausoleum, because Angie had twice said she never wanted to be put in the ground. After determining that Gethsemane Cemetery Mausoleum in New Hope was the right location, I spoke with the cemetery director about our "needs" and that the crypt would be needed soon. After the meeting, I had driven the twenty-five minutes back to the hospital, looking at the homes decorated with bright Christmas lights that blurred through my tears.

Angie's "treasure chest," from a casket manufacturer in Minneapolis, was a beautiful bronze casket custom painted pink for Angie. The following message was embroidered in the satin of the inner lid:

> Sleep tight and have
> sweet, sweet dreams,
> Daddy's Little Princess and
> Mama Bear's Baby Bear
> and Best Friend.
> We love you, and the three
> of us will be together now,
> always and forever.
> Daddy and Mama Bear

DESPITE HAVING ALREADY selected the mausoleum site and casket, the days leading up to the funeral were still busy. We met with Fr. Tim twice to plan the service. We selected songs and readings. Fr. Tim chose the message. Linda wrote an obituary for publication, and I wrote the eulogy. Both were composed in the form of a love letter to Angie. We worked together to find the words to describe what we wanted to say. I wrote what Linda and I felt: "We believe that the angels carried you on their wings to be cradled in the arms of God forever." We thought Angela would make a perfect angel.

Dick and Jeanne Johnson helped us plan a reception to be held after the interment. We didn't want the occasion to be a "typical" church basement affair. We decided to hold our commemorative gathering at The Women's Club in Minneapolis. The beautiful old mansion evoked the dignity befitting a solemn day of grief. We hired a pianist and chose Angela's favorite foods, including "Dad's" barbecued hamburgers, chicken fingers, quesadillas, and lots of fruit.

The evenings and nights prior to the funeral were the most difficult. Too tired to do more preparation, Linda and I sat together staring at the television. We could not wait to fall asleep so the pain would subside for a while and the awful memories of the previous months could drift out of our consciousness until we awoke—usually every hour or two. The morning light provided some exhilaration, enough to accomplish the unspeakably hurtful tasks of the day. What I remember most of that time was not the details of the tasks and planning, but rather the sheer emptiness I felt—as though all breath had been sucked out of me.

We called February 10, 2003, the day of Angie's funeral, a day of celebration. We were "celebrating" Angie's magnificent life. But for Linda and me, the day was another experience of shock and grief. Well-meaning friends and family told us that, in time, our shock and grief would gradually dissipate. I still question that assumption. Though others may have been able to celebrate Angie's life, my thoughts that day were dominated by the countless joys and experiences cystic fibrosis had stolen from her.

I think we expected to feel more of a sense of finality. Many family members and friends present knew little of the past months and the enormity of the tragic events. Linda and I had to retell and relive the nightmares many times. February 10, 2003, was a day to survive.

Fortunately, the day was focused on Angie, so laughter and fond memories were also shared. I was happy to see so many of her high school classmates. Angie's friends J.D., Marcia, and Steve served as pallbearers along with her godparents Judi and Michael, cousins Tracy and Brian, and her uncle Bill. Her boyfriend Josh sat with our family. Linda and I were touched that Darvin from 4D came to Angela's funeral. His wife was still in the hospital, but a work associate of mine had volunteered to pick up Darvin and make sure he had rides to and from the funeral and reception.

The service began with a brief prayer at the entry of the church near the Baptismal Font. The sound system played "When a Child Is Born" by Kenny Rogers. The Mass included several readings; Dick Johnson read the eulogy/love letter we wrote to Angie. Other songs played were Bette Midler's "Wind Beneath My Wings" and "My Heart Will Go On" from the movie *Titanic*, a favorite of Angie's.

We sang hymns, including "Amazing Grace," "Softly and Tenderly" (my mother's favorite), and "The Old Rugged Cross" (a favorite of Linda's mother). "Softly and Tenderly" had been sung at my brother's funeral in 1966, my father's in 1967, and my mother's only a year earlier. What memories the hymn invoked for me!

After the Mass, the caravan of cars stretched for miles along the fifteen or so miles to the mausoleum at Gethsemane. Linda and I rode in the backseat as Dick drove. Jeanne sat next to him in the front seat. As we sat, dazed by grief, Jeanne turned around in the car and, as only Jeanne could do, lifted the entire mood for a brief moment.

She said, "I am going in for plastic surgery tomorrow."

We all went, "Huh?"

Apparently one of Linda's relatives had come up to Jeanne and asked her if she was my mother. All four of us laughed hard for several moments, releasing some of the tension of the day.

THE ONLY SONG PLAYED at the interment was "Fly," by Celine Dion. "Fly" has special meaning in the CF community because Celine Dion wrote the song about her niece who passed away as a result of cystic fibrosis.

Fr. Steve LaCanne led the service at the cemetery. As the hospital priest, he had lived the ICU experience with us. Those eighty-six days had profoundly affected his life. He was one of so many who prayed and hoped and waited for a miracle to heal Angie. Father Steve had suggested to us that perhaps we already had our miracle—the gift of Angela and our wonderful chance to have and care for her for almost twenty-two years. Linda and I appreciated his wisdom. Angela was and will always be our miracle.

The reception at The Women's Club was beautiful. As the evening wore on, no one wanted to leave. My brother Dennis had come from Big Rapids, Michigan, with his wife, Cheryl, and their four children, Melissa, Rachel, Eric, and Amanda. Linda's sister Mary had flown in from Denver. Even as we gathered together, though, my own heart was back at Gethsemane with my little girl. Linda and I could not glance at each other across the room without tears welling in our eyes. Occasionally, the pianist unwittingly played a song from the service or a special song for Angie, Linda, or me that served as further "triggers" of powerful emotion.

Most of the guests left by 8:00 P.M. However, family members and a few close friends stayed until 11:00 P.M., engaged in sad conversation and nostalgic remembrances. The mood of the evening was quiet, making the voice shouting in my head even louder—*Where is the rage? She did not deserve what happened to her! I want Angela alive and with us!*

But I kept those thoughts inside.

ONE OF THE MOST TOUCHING STORIES I heard that day was from my good friend of thirty years, John Fallon. He and I were fraternity brothers in college, best friends, and groomsmen in each other's weddings. Now we were golf partners and cherished friends. John had a talent for bringing fun and laughter to any gathering. During our eighty-six ICU days, he had been a visitor once or twice a week. He brought the occasional bottle of "good" scotch to share with everyone in 4D. During each visit, John had a way of pouring light on the dismal gloom of our daily struggle.

John had not been aware of our final decision to let Angie go on February 6, 2003. He had arrived at the hospital after she died. He found the 4D lounge and Angela's hospital bed empty. A nurse told him what had happened. At the reception, John told me how sad he had been and how he had gone out to a bar that night by himself and cried. The image of my dear friend alone in a bar, grieving the death of my daughter, Angie, was seared in my mind.

THE DAY OF ANGIE'S FUNERAL ended with hugs of love and best wishes for everyone. During a time of such sadness, being surrounded by family and friends brought soothing comfort.

I believe many people thought Linda and I would ultimately feel some relief that the nightmare was over. But the nightmare did not end that day. Jeanne Johnson left me with the most insightful comment of the day, which stayed in my mind as Linda and I drove home from Angie's funeral, holding hands in silence.

Jeanne said, "You will laugh with others, and you will cry alone."

The crying had just begun.

For the next several days Linda and I were exhausted. We shed many tears, alone and together. Life would never again be the same. How could anything be the same? As I moved about our community, grocery shopping or performing other necessary tasks, happy people, many with their children, went about their business, shopping for Valentine's Day cards or gifts. They behaved so normally. I again thought of Frank Deford's book, *Alex: The Life of a Child*. Deford, a *Sports Illustrated* writer, lost his daughter Alex at age eight to cystic fibrosis. His book was the first I had read about cystic fibrosis and the loss of a child. I had read Deford's book several times over the years and once again in the months before Angie died. In one section of the book, Deford spoke about his interactions with the outside world as his daughter was dying and after her death. He spoke of similar observations of people. In a large city, of course, people go about their daily lives, oblivious to the most momentous tragedy that may have happened to someone passing in the street. Like Frank Deford, I wanted to scream, "How can you be so happy and act so normal when the most beautiful girl in the world has just died! My heart is broken! Can't you see that?"

But, of course, rather than drop to the ground and cry out until the pain subsided, I, like Deford, moved forward, trying to behave as though life went on as normal. If doing so had been in Angela's best interest, I would have lived in the 4D lounge forever, for I could still have held her hand, exercised her arms and legs, and rubbed her little nose and forehead.

J.D.'S GRANDPARENTS HAD taken loving care of Angie's little dog. A few days after the funeral, Torrance came home. Linda held Torrance in her arms in the car. My wife had not grown up with dogs and did not think she'd want to live with a dog. But from the time Angie brought Torrance home to stay, Linda had fallen in love with her just as I had. Now Linda's outpouring of love reached a new level as she cared for Torrance, knowing that was what our daughter would have wanted. The little white dog was a living, bright-eyed, loving part of Angie.

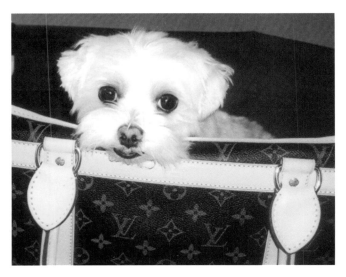

WITHIN DAYS OF ANGELA'S PASSING, I wrote a letter to Arthur Roy in Wyoming, telling him of the events of the preceding weeks. After receiving my letter, Amanda called to tell me her brother Travis had died on February 7, 2003, only twelve hours after Angela passed away. Amanda told me her father could not speak to me by phone, but he would write a letter soon. Within a couple of weeks, I received his letter:

Dear Don and Linda,

I admire your courage in writing your letter to me, at a time of such sorrow for all of us. I only too well understand your devastation. The old adage "time heals everything" offers little solace at a time like this. "Time" is so relative.

My brother, Tom, was someone I deeply loved and respected. He was the last of our family to be taken by CF just over fourteen years ago, and I still weep at his memory.

His case was different than yours. He needed an immediate heart/lung transplant or go on a ventilator and wait and hope for a match. He then called me and asked me if I would come to Laramie, Wyoming, and hold him while he died. He would not put his wife and two young kids through the agony you and Linda just endured.

Fourteen years ago his chance for a transplant was nearly zero, and the CF had so ravaged the rest of his body, it was, in his mind, only prolonging the inevitable. I so loved and admired his courage.

He was my younger brother by three years, and I did not want to let him go. Despite his lifelong illness he was the happiest, funniest, full-of-life person I have ever known. So I did what he asked and gathered the family and in three long days and nights he finally gave up his life. I had my head on his chest and his arm around my shoulder and heard his heart beat for the last time.

So you see, my dear friends in sorrow, I feel your pain, even clear out here in Wyoming. As for my beloved son Travis, I am sure that Amanda has let you know that he left us on February 7th.

I thought I had suffered devastation before in my life, having lost my parents, two sisters and two brothers. They were great losses but now I know the true meaning of devastation.

Travis was so much more than my son! He was my kindred spirit! My friend! I loved him more than my own life! Travis and I talked of his disease as a series of hurdles and options. As long as he had one more option he still had hope.

On the night of January 29th, I got down on my knees in front of his wheelchair, took his hands in mine and told him the MRI was very bad and that he had no more options. He replied "No more options? Please, Dad, just one more option!"

He sobbed in my arms and in the arms of his wife for a few minutes and then sat up and said, "Well, I guess that is that. When can I go home?" We took him home the next day, and the rest is history.

For his memorial service, I did his eulogy; his mom added a part, as did each of his siblings. I cried the morning he died. I did his forty-minute eulogy without a single tear. I finally, thank God, broke down on February 21st, two weeks after he died and cried for days and now weeks.

We hold so much of our emotions in as a show of strength for our children, and for such a long time, that when the emotional dam does break it is a virtual flood of tears. As for "time heals all things" I am not sure I agree. I believe that God expects us, with his help, to grow spiritually strong enough to bear the burden he has given us. I do not believe any parent can heal from a loss of this magnitude. Rather, I believe lying quietly under the surface will remain the pain and sorrow but also the love and happiness, which ebb and flow with each memory of the child we have lost.

I have spent weeks writing thank-you cards to so many compassionate people who came to our aid in our time of great sorrow that at times I feel as though my words are simply my soul bleeding onto paper.

I wish for each of you peace, serenity, and spiritual growth and ask that you place your sorrows in God's hands and allow him to lessen your burden.

Yours in sorrow,

Arthur Roy

God bless Arthur Roy and so many others we came to know in the 4D lounge, "The Family Room," during the eighty-six days we endured there. We met many other loving families—like the family who saved the best couches on the fourth floor for Linda and me because they believed we needed them more than someone there for only a night or two. Their wife and mother passed away while waiting for a heart transplant. There was the wife and two bright sons of a Russian man who was dying from a brain hemorrhage. We sat talking with them in the lounge late at night during Angela's final weeks. They remained after we left. People we scarcely knew stopped outside Angie's room to say a prayer. "The Family Room" saw countless prayers of substance. Linda and I will forever carry in our hearts the memory of so many strangers with whom we shared so much, for so long.

FOOTPRINTS IN THE SAND

One night I dreamed I was walking along the beach with the Lord.
Many scenes from my life flashed across the sky.
In each scene I noticed footprints in the sand.
Sometimes there were two sets of footprints;
other times there were one set of footprints.
This bothered me because I noticed
that during the low periods of my life,
when I was suffering from anguish, sorrow, or defeat,
I could see only one set of footprints.
So I said to the Lord,
"You promised me Lord,
that if I followed you,
you would walk with me always.
But I have noticed that during the most trying periods of my life
there have only been one set of footprints in the sand.
Why, when I needed you most, you have not been there for me?"
The Lord replied,
"The times when you have seen only one set of footprints in the sand,
is when I carried you."

Mary Stevenson

PART FIVE

FINDING
AN
IN-BETWEEN

Returning to work was difficult for me, but so was remaining isolated in full-time mourning. Linda and I badly needed to find some normality after months of horror. Her family was a source of great comfort to her as she battled the heartache. A particular source of comfort for me came from the sage advice of a man and friend whom I respected so much, Bob Sparboe. Bob was about seventy years old, a huge success in business and finance, a man of great intellectual curiosity, and a fountain of wisdom. Twenty-five years earlier he had lost a son to a lifelong illness. His experience included an extensive period when his son was in intensive care, ultimately resulting in his son's death. Bob had been forced to set up his business and life in an ICU. We understood where each other had been. We talked about our experiences and of the promises of our faith about eternity. We talked of indescribable loss and heartbreak, and so much more. We spoke of how one can transform a tragedy into something positive for others.

When I asked Bob to share with me how he got through the loss of his son and later his wife, he said the only action he found effective was "going back to work" and "doing good works for others." Bob stressed the importance of service and using every experience as an opportunity to make a positive contribution to the world. He had printed his message on a greeting card:

> One of life's most valuable talents is the ability to drive positive energy and direction from adversity as well as from success.
>
> Carpe Diem—Seize the Day!

JUST AS THE INTENSITY OF ACTIVITY and interactions with so many others was winding down for Linda and me, I received a call from Renee Stewart. She was a writer who had been touched by the obituary Linda had written for Angie. She wanted to write an article about Angie for the *Eden Prairie News*. Renee requested an interview. I told her I'd think about her idea and call her back.

Linda and I discussed whether I should do the interview. She had been feeling grateful that our day-to-day life had been, to some extent, calmer. Her first thought was to protect Angela's privacy. Linda didn't think Angela would want that kind of attention. I agreed that I would never want to betray Angela, but I pointed out that she had been a cheerleader. She was not an introvert. She was an outgoing, loving and energetic soul. I added, "There must be an in-between."

Bob Sparboe's philosophy of creating something positive out of adversity was in my mind a week later when I called Renee Stewart and agreed to the interview. I had decided that sharing Angie's story was a way of paying tribute to our brave daughter as well as educating others about the devastation of cystic fibrosis.

The beautifully written article, "Remembering Their Little Angel," was published on March 20, 2003, on the front page of the *Eden Prairie News*. The story featured photos of Angie, Linda, and me. For a few days after the article's publication, Linda doubted my decision to go public with Angie's story. But after a short while, she saw the article as the loving tribute I had intended.

Slowly, days and weeks passed. Yet, not one day passed that thoughts of Angie didn't bring tears. Some days the tears flowed freely. There were days when I just wished the pain would go away. Yet, I didn't really want the pain to leave, for missing her was one way Angie stayed in my life. Linda and I were often asked how we were doing. We responded with the usual "fine." But, in truth, living with a broken heart was extremely difficult, for our hearts bled every day.

My desire to do more in Angie's honor was not yet satisfied. I began to explore options for establishing a foundation in Angie's memory. Others came forward to honor Angie as well. Some of my clients and several members of our family wanted to make contributions of various sorts in Angie's name. By May we had a defined mission for the foundation and a partner, the Minnesota Community Foundation, to assist us in meeting our goals in Angie's name. Around this same time, Linda and I were invited to meet with representatives from the Cystic Fibrosis Foundation. The entire foundation board had been moved by Linda's obituary for Angela, as well as the article that appeared in the *Eden Prairie News*. As a result, the organization representatives wanted our blessing to rename the annual award given to the person who made the greatest impact toward the goal of finding a cure for cystic fibrosis. The new name for the honor was to be the *Angela Warner Friend of the Foundation Award*.

The recipient that year was to be Dr. Warren Warwick. Few people had been so tirelessly devoted to the fight against CF, or been responsible for so many scientific and clinical breakthroughs to help CF patients. He had dedicated his life to the care of CF patients and to curing the disease. My respect for Dr. Warwick had not diminished in all the years he had assisted, directly or indirectly, in Angie's care. Linda and I remained particularly grateful that he helped us survive our last Christmas Eve with Angie.

The following November at the *2003 Breath of Life Gala* sponsored by the Minnesota Chapter of the Cystic Fibrosis Foundation, I had the opportunity to tell the story of Dr. Warwick's Christmas Eve with us. Linda and I were asked to present the first *Angela Warner Friend of the Foundation Award* to Dr. Warwick. In addition to the award presentation, a remembrance of Angela in the form of a video with pictures of her was presented. The background music was a recording of "Wind Beneath My Wings."

THE FIRST TIME I RETURNED to Laguna after Angie's death was October 2004. Linda wasn't ready to make the trip yet. Going back to the Surf and Sand was an emotional experience. I took along one of my favorite pictures of Angela in a solid glass frame. Linda sent along with me the poem "Footprints in the Sand" and a note, telling me that Angie would be at my side always as I walked the beach. As soon as I entered my room at the Surf and Sand and looked out at the sparkling Pacific Ocean, the truth was clear: Angie's presence would always be here for me. The waves were crashing on the beach as I took my first walk on the sand in the afternoon. The little footprints I saw as I walked along the edge of the water brought flashbacks of seeing Angie's footprints as a child beside mine, or often in front of mine, as she ran ahead to play in the waves.

That day the surf was strong enough to produce a heavy mist that rolled off the surf line onto the beach. The ethereal effect matched my feelings, as I walked through the hazy air and felt the hot sun and the waves spraying my legs. The beach was almost empty; the footprints must have been from earlier in the day.

While daytime walks for Angie and me together were commonplace and fun because of the sunshine and playfulness, my first nighttime walk without her triggered the most emotion for me.

As I stepped out on the sand that first night, the only lights that shone on the beach were from the Surf and Sand and the homes along the coast. I walked in the darkness alone, remembering so many of those conversations with my daughter through the years. We spoke of how we appreciated the beauty of this place and the enormity, depth of mystery, and vastness of the sea. No matter how long our own lives, they were only short stories in the history of the world. When Angela was small, I think those were my messages to her about my mortality relative to hers; but without saying so, the roles reversed to some extent in later years.

Our nighttime walks were the times Angie and I shared our thoughts about the universe and eternity and how the endless waves had washed ashore for billions of years, that the stars we saw were really as they were millions of years ago because the light took that long to travel so far to reach Earth. Together, Angie and I were awed by the starry heavens above us.

But now as I walked along that same beach in the quiet darkness and looked up at the endless number of stars in the sky, I realized that Angie now had the answers, and I was still left with the questions. I cried again and again, for I should have been the one leading the way for Angela in finding the real answers to many of our questions about life, the universe, death, and eternity. Linda always identified one star in a sky as Angela's, but the entire sky was Angela's now. She was already in the inconceivable and unimaginable place, so why not trust that she could now comprehend these mysteries?

For her, most of all, but also for Linda and me, I wished that Angela had had the opportunity to live a long life on this Earth. I wished she could have experienced all life's pleasures and joys before leaving forever. In my tears were sadness and anger at the unfairness of fighting cystic fibrosis all those years, the degrading experiences during the days leading to surgery, and the eighty days in intensive care, leading to the decision that letting her go was a form of a gift from us to her. Was our choice a gift? Only the answers to the questions Angie and I talked about on our nightly walks on the beach could provide a respite to my tears.

I walked along the shoreline every night during that first visit back. Angie's picture sat on a table, looking at the ocean. I felt her presence then, and I feel her now each time I return to my, that is, our, beloved Laguna Beach.

There is sacredness in tears.
They are not the mark of weakness, but of power.
They speak more eloquently than 10,000 tongues.
They are the messengers of overwhelming grief, of deep contrition,
and of unspeakable love.

– Washington Irving

LINDA RETURNED TO LAGUNA with me for the first time in August 2005, two and a half years after Angie died. The trip generated a surge of emotion. Linda was not a nighttime beach walker, but she had her own special memories with Angela: walking the streets of Laguna, window-shopping and regular shopping, talking and laughing on their visits to Fashion Island and the South Coast Mall in Costa Mesa.

A hard part for Linda was our drive down the flower-lined streets of Laguna Beach, entering the town from the north on the Pacific Coast Highway. She grabbed my hand tightly and tears ran down her cheeks as we drove. More difficult for her was the first time we walked into our room at the Surf and Sand, looking clear through to the ocean. Angie always ran straight to the deck, and pushed the doors open to go outside to feel the ocean breezes. Then within moments she'd be pulling our arms to go "hit" the beach.

Linda and I stood on the deck with our arms entwined, each of us remembering so much about Angela, and the countless times she stood on that same spot over the years. Angie's childlike enthusiasm always appeared brightest when the ocean was at her feet. That is, except at night, when our conversations turned to the serious and wondrous—the inconceivable and unimaginable.

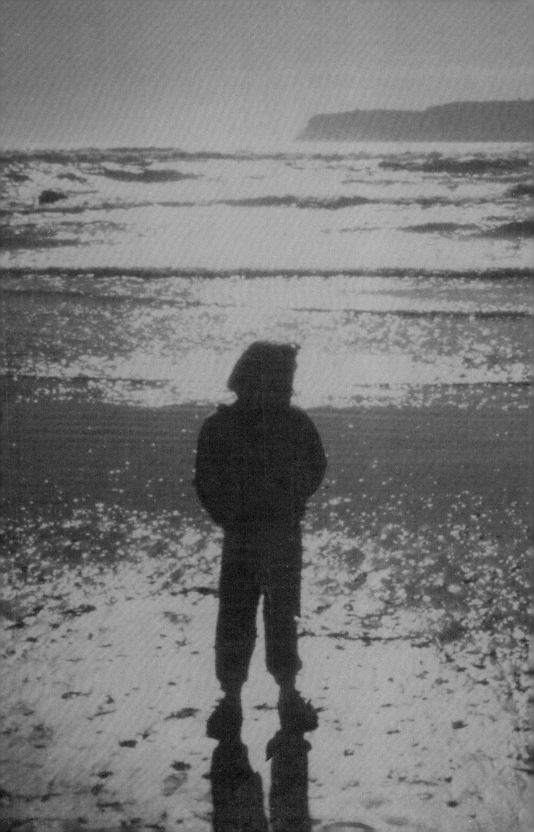

EPILOGUE:
LIVING ON
WITH
A
BROKEN
HEART

About one year after Angela's death, a car accident occurred west of the Twin Cities, killing three sisters on their way to their brother's wedding rehearsal. All the local news media covered the story, and everyone was talking about the tragedy. During a breakfast conversation with my friend Dick Johnson, he asked me what I would say to the parents of those three girls if I had the opportunity. My answer came quickly and with clarity after one year of my own heartsickness.

I said, "I would tell them how sorry I was for their daughters and for them. Theirs was a horrible tragedy, and despite what people may tell them, they will never get over or recover from what happened to their children; they will only learn to survive their loss. They may learn to live with a broken heart, but life will never be the same. Most importantly, I would say that no matter how horrible they feel now and going forward, their feelings are valid. The pain is real. And, finally, I would affirm their hope, a hope beyond hope, that one day they will be able to reunite with their children."

Dick's eyes met mine for a long moment with a "you are speaking the truth" look. I thought I was.

C.S. LEWIS WROTE IN *A Grief Observed* that prior to his wife's death, he found it quite easy to pray for those he referred to as "the other dead." He recognized he was somewhat unconcerned as to whether others went to Heaven, or nowhere, or even hell. He simply did not have a compelling need for an absolute answer to the question of where our loved ones go after their death. Upon the death of his wife, Joy, whom he loved more profoundly than he ever imagined possible, he *had to know* the truth. He could not pray for her as he had "the other dead." The question of eternal life was now the most important single question to be answered. He did not need to know out of concern for his own fate; he needed the answer for *Joy*.

When I read the words of C.S. Lewis, they crystallized my own thoughts. I can live with what happened to Angie only because of the glorious eternal life our faith promises. I am able to speak to her and pray for her. These are now the most meaningful prayers of my life. I was raised a Christian, to have faith in God. I hadn't given much thought to the questions: *What if none of it is true? What if there is nothing after our death?*

After Angie's death, those questions became the most important questions imaginable for me, too. They are important to me personally, but Angie is the one I am most concerned about. I want her to be in that "better place" that C.S. Lewis describes as "inconceivable and unimaginable." In my unscientific opinion, I believe that even the strongest believers have at least shreds of doubt, and the most adamant nonbelievers harbor a trace of hope in an afterlife. The rest of us lie on a continuum between the two extremes.

Linda and I have often been told how unimaginable our pain must be to have lost Angela. The pain is imaginable because Linda and I and many other parents endure it. We have frequently been asked if we have "gotten over" Angie's death or even if we "feel better" now. I recognize how well meaning such questions may be, but I usually want to respond with, "We did not have the flu. We lost the most important person in the world to us, and we will never 'get over' the loss, nor do I want to 'get over' losing Angie."

I once heard a counselor compare the loss of a child to having both legs amputated. Life goes on but is forever altered. He described these losses as survivable tragedies. However, I find the analogy of lost limbs completely useless. I would trade *all* my limbs without hesitation to have Angie still in my life. Without a second thought, I would sacrifice my own life for hers if doing so meant she could have even a few more years.

I have yet to hear an analogy that accurately reflects the feelings surrounding the death of a child. I know of no counseling capable of reducing the heartache. Does the parent of a lost child ever find *peace*? Some satisfaction comes from doing good works, not allowing the loss to be without meaning or significance. Good works, however, do not provide peace.

Charles Dickens asked, "And can it be that in a world so full and busy, the loss of one weak creature makes a void in any heart, so wide and deep that nothing but the width and depth of eternity can fill it up?" Within his question Dickens identifies the depth of the loss of a child and also provides insight into how such a loss is survivable, how a *degree* of peace is possible. He identifies eternity as the only thing deep and wide enough to be that source of peace for a grieving parent.

The loss of my child is only endured because I am learning to live with a broken heart. The wound, or void, is too deep and wide to be healed in this lifetime. The grieving never ends. The pain is always present. I understood what C.S. Lewis meant when he wrote about his wife, "Her absence is like the sky, spread over everything."

For a short time after Angie's death, I was able to grieve and share the pain publicly. But, in time, most of my pain and grief had to be private, as the rest of the world moved on. I have looked into the eyes of other grieving parents but I can only do so briefly, for in those eyes I see a broken heart that is forever. Some days bring less bleeding, but the wound does not heal. And, even years later, the bleeding reappears and sometimes does not relent for days or weeks. I am learning to live with the wound that is wide and deep but not entirely healed. Jeanne Johnson's words on the day of Angie's funeral still ring true: *You will laugh with others and you will cry alone.*

As time passed, I was aware and often reminded that others had moved on. Fewer references to Angie were made in my presence. I sometimes wondered if others thought about or remembered her. My personal assistant, Emily Schaefbauer, had been with me for a few years prior to Angela's death and was about the same age as Angela. Emily had witnessed much of what Linda and I endured in surviving our daughter's death. She wrote a letter to us for Christmas 2005, almost three years after Angie died. The letter set to rest some of my wonderings. Linda and I were touched by Emily's depth of insight into our many unspoken thoughts.

December 23, 2005

Dear Don & Linda,

Two Christmases ago, I read a passage in a book that I thought was just beautiful. I was Christmas shopping at the time, and intended to buy it and give it to you. Somehow, it wasn't in any of my bags when I got home. I went back to the store where I had found it (and many other bookstores as well) with no luck. I couldn't recall the title, and no one at any of the bookstores knew which book I was talking about.

Even though I forgot how the passage went, the sentiment of it always comes to mind when I think of the two of you dealing with different holidays and dates of significance. Any given year for you must seem like a minefield. Holidays are fine for people who haven't experienced a devastating loss in their family. For those who have, they just seem like another painful reminder of that loss.

A couple of weeks ago I was in the same store where I first saw the book that got away. I was thinking about it (i.e., kicking myself) when the gift enclosed fell on my head. One of the store clerks was rearranging some things on a shelf above me and accidentally knocked it down. Can you believe that I searched high and low for years for this saying, and then one day, while I was thinking about it again, it just fell on my head? The store clerk was so apologetic, she couldn't understand why I was thanking her for dropping this on me.

I took it as a sign that I needed to finish the letter I should have sent a long time ago.

I don't know where to start describing all of the feelings and emotions I have had for the past couple of years in regards to having been witness to your tragedy. First and foremost, throughout this all I have come to know that you both have many people that love you greatly and are concerned with your well being. You are surrounded by many who care deeply for you. I have felt angry at God on your and your daughter's behalf for having to live with the remarkable unfairness in life. I have felt guilty for being young and healthy in your presence. I don't know if I could be that bigger person and not resent every young person who didn't know what it was like to have to struggle on a constant basis for health like your own daughter had to. I have sincerely felt my heart break for you both.

I have experienced the loss of family members, but certainly the loss I know is in no way comparable to the loss you have endured. Obviously there is no comparison. I know that what you have lived through is something which no one else could ever understand unless they themselves had been through it as well. People may sympathize, but only those who have walked that road can ever have a true understanding of what it is to live through a loss of that proportion. This is one of the reasons that I haven't been forthcoming in sharing or expressing the sorrow I feel for you. Since I don't truly know what it must be like for you to go on in life — nor do I have a real conceptual understanding of the diligence and dedication it took to keep Angela healthy while you were raising her — I have been very internal. What right do I have to think I could possibly understand? Please do not take any reclusiveness on my part as lack of compassion. I, along with everyone else, certainly wish that I could have made things different for you and that there had been a different outcome. I wish you didn't have to experience every Mother's Day and Father's Day and Thanksgiving and Christmas without your daughter. I wish I had the answers to all of the profound questions in life as to why things are the way they are that no one really has.

Your loss is so profound, so intensely significant that I know in my heart no complete healing is possible. I know that your pain will remain for a lifetime, and yet I'm sure Angela, as much as she loved you, would not want you to feel sadness. This must be one of the most tragic ironies of life. Besides, you will be with her again soon enough. I think you do her great honor to make a sincere attempt at happiness during the time you have left to live.

After all of this, I hope I haven't said anything to offend you. Also, please forgive me for the times I have appeared to be insensitive (and I know there have been times). In my opinion and experience, unless someone lives it, they cannot understand it. Please know that I have certainly never intentionally meant to be callous.

Finally, I want to let you know how very shocked and surprised I was to have been asked by you to serve as a successor chair member for Angela's scholarship fund at the U. Since portraying emotion in person is not my strong suit, I will say that I am honored that you consider me fit to do so. After everything I have learned from Angela, it is honoring to have the opportunity to serve her memory. You have my word that when the day comes, I will be conscientious to the fund and the goings on. Please rest assured that I will remain aware always. I am truly humbled by the opportunity to help, and am always available to help if you need me.

Thank you for everything. I wish you both the best, always.

Emily

Along with Emily's letter was a gift of a silver angel ornament inscribed with:

> *Perhaps they are not stars in the sky*
> *but rather openings where our loved ones*
> *shine down to let us know they are happy.*

LOOKING AT THE SILVER ANGEL, I again felt the love for my angel, my Angela, filling the starry sky. Albert Einstein said, "Two things inspire me to awe—the starry heavens above and the moral universe within." To my human mind, the infinity and order of the universe is still incomprehensible and unimaginable. From the vast starry heavens and depth of the ocean to the grains of sand and the complexity of the atom, how can I argue that a superior mind or spirit did not construct the laws of the universe? The morality placed in each of us to care for others in our lives and for humanity in general—through our good works and our love—gives life beauty and meaning. Such morality is a universal evidence of God.

Not a day passes that my heart is not saddened for a time as my mind is focused on Angela, but Linda and I have been fortunate to remain surrounded by those who have cared for us: loving family, old friends, and new friends. The love and the laughter we share is a tonic that is strong and brings us great joy. Particularly gratifying has been the relationships we have been able to maintain with those who were close to Angela. J.D. continues to be a devoted friend whom we love. We thoroughly enjoy frequent dinners together. As he wrote of his relationship with Angie, we continue to be there for each other.

Josh has also remained close to us. In 2004, Linda and I became business partners with him through the purchase of a Quizno's restaurant in Plymouth, Minnesota, that he manages. We named our corporation ABW Enterprises, LLC. Josh often called Angie by her initials, ABW. Josh is far more than a business partner to us; he is a special friend who will always have our love.

LINDA AND I REMAIN HOPEFUL that our lives here on Earth continue to be filled with love, laughter, and purpose. For at least a year after Angie's death, the latter two seemed unlikely to return, and the former seemed less important with our child gone. But, Angie had shown us how to love and blessed us with the opportunity to love her. As a result, love is still abundant in our lives. Laughter and joy are constants again, and we are grateful. As for purpose, Angie left us a legacy of love that is a powerful inspiration.

For Linda and me, comfort and peace come from our faith that promises us that Angela is in Heaven, and Linda and I will reunite with her in time. I cannot imagine life without the possibility.

> Love ... bears all things, believes all things,
> hopes all things, endures all things.
> Love never ends ...
>
> 1 Corinthians 13:7-8 RSV

I love you, Angie, with all my heart. Until I see you again,
Dad

ANGIE'S LEGACY OF LOVE

February 6, 2003, changed life forever for Linda and me. We lost our precious child, the love of our lives. Nothing could ever again be the same. The horror of that day and the eighty-five preceding days were etched in our memories. But prior to those days were twenty-one years and 247 days that created meaning and guided the course of our lives. Angela was the one who taught us how to love *completely*. With her genuine and pure heart, she inspired her parents to be better people. As advocates for our child in a relentless fight against cystic fibrosis, we learned to be advocates for her happiness and for her future. This was the role we cherished most in life.

As I sat through the many lonely hours in the ICU holding Angie's hands, exercising her arms and legs or rubbing her forehead or nose, I prayed for her. I reflected on how I did not want to relinquish the job of advocate for this person I loved beyond imagination. I saw during those dark days that my life to a great degree would be dedicated either to her care—for if she survived, her recovery would be long and difficult—or to creating an enduring legacy in her name. Linda and I continue to be her advocates, carrying on the "business" of Angie's life.

Most of us have the opportunity to create our own legacy through our children, grandchildren, our vocation, our good works, and gifts of our time, talent, and resources *during* our lives. Angie certainly left an indelible mark on those with whom she shared her life, but how does a twenty-one-year-old person complete a legacy when her life has been cut short? I am committed to fulfilling Angie's legacy. Linda and I spend much of our lives doing just that. We will do what we can to assure Angie's story and her brave spirit is remembered.

The abundant unconditional love Angela bestowed on Linda and me and her family and friends was the inheritance she left us. Linda and I only hope she is pleased with the projects we have initiated (so far) in her memory:

- The Angela Warner Foundation
- The Angela Warner Children's Memorial and Prayer Garden
- The Angela Warner Friend of the Foundation Award
- The Angela Brooke Warner CF Scholarship Endowment Fund
- *Walks on the Beach with Angie: A Father's Story of Love*

The Angela Warner Foundation

The initial purpose of *The Angela Warner Foundation* was to provide scholarships and grants for medical research focused on finding a cure for cystic fibrosis. After further exploration into philanthropic options, Linda and I decided to expand the scope of the foundation's mission. We established a donor-advised fund through the Minnesota Community Foundation with an arrangement that offers simplicity and ease of administration, while meeting our gifting goals. *The Angela Warner Foundation* was established on May 23, 2003.

The Angela Warner Foundation supports a scholarship program at Angie's alma mater, Eden Prairie High School, and provides financial support to the Cystic Fibrosis Foundation to help in its pursuit of a cure for cystic fibrosis. Linda and I continue to seek opportunities to expand the activities of the foundation with more initiatives that exemplify Angie's generous heart.

Angela Warner Foundation
C/o Donald A. Warner,
801 Twelve Oaks Center Drive, Suite 826,
Wayzata, MN 55391

www.angelawarnerfoundation.org

The Angela Warner Children's Memorial and Prayer Garden

I frequently visit the mausoleum chapel at Gethsemane Cemetery where Angie was laid to rest. In the weeks after she passed away, I visited daily and prayed for my darling daughter. Our family's crypts are adjacent to a large glass door and floor-to-ceiling window, facing west. The afternoon sun shines brightly on Angie's photograph and a flower arrangement that adorns her resting place. About thirty feet from the door is a grove of pine trees with open acreage beyond. For the first year or two, I looked out at the pine trees and thought the space called for something special. One day in 2005 an idea hit me. The grove of pine trees was the perfect environment for a memorial to Angela and a prayer garden for other parents who have endured the horror and pain of losing a child.

I approached the executive director of The Catholic Cemeteries, John Cherek, with my idea. He had also lost a daughter when she was about Angie's age. For three years, Linda, and I worked closely with John, Dave Kemp, and others at The Catholic Cemeteries with a goal to create an extraordinary environment capable of providing families with peace and a place to mourn and remember. After much hard work, *The Angela Warner Children's Memorial and Prayer Garden* became a reality.

The garden has five primary features. First is a large granite wall imprinted with a poem Linda and I wrote in 2005.

LAMENT FOR A CHILD

We come here to mourn and remember
the children who have gone before us.

We seek peace but it is elusive.

We hold sacred all the remembrances of those
who were the sunshine of our lives.
We were blessed to have them touch our souls forever.

Our love for them is wider than the sky and deeper than the ocean.
They returned such love unconditionally.

We shall remember the precious children
for they danced upon the earth and are now Eternal Angels.

Through Amazing Grace we shall one day gather with them and the Saints
at that beautiful river near the throne of God.

Written in Memory of Angela Warner
by Donald and Linda Warner
2005

ANGIE'S LOVE OF DOLPHINS and the ocean inspired a pool and fountain with large rocks and a bronze dolphin family emerging from the water. The sound of running water provides a tranquil backdrop for three monuments that stand almost ten feet high. Bronze angels rest atop granite columns. Each angel has a theme and message.

The dedication and memorial to Angela is on the granite below *The Angel of the Resurrection* with a small collage of pictures of Angie etched in bronze. The angel is releasing a butterfly.

THE ANGEL OF THE RESURRECTION

Sets us free to eternal life with God.
A butterfly lights beside us like a sunbeam . . . and for a brief
Moment its glory and beauty belong to this world . . .
But then it flies on again, and although we wish it could
Have stayed, we are so thankful to have seen it at all.

The Angel of Creation signifies that God gave us the blessing of life. The angel holds a conch shell suggesting that blessings flow like water from the seashell. The shell was molded from a conch shell we brought back from the Surf and Sand in Laguna when Linda and I went there together in August 2005 for the first time after Angie's death.

THE ANGEL OF CREATION

Pours forth all of God's blessings
Abundantly upon us . . .
As water from the sea flows endlessly
From the shell . . .

Our children were born to us as gifts
From God . . .
They were treasured and cherished
In life . . .

God now holds them in the palm
Of His hand

The Angel of the Breath of Life is dedicated to those who have lost the battle with cystic fibrosis. The message emphasizes the continued need for work to find a cure.

THE ANGEL OF THE BREATH OF LIFE

Reminds us God is the source
Of all life . . .

God breathed life into our children
So we may come to know
Love and joy
As a foretaste of being one with Him
Forever in the kingdom of Heaven.

Gethsemane Cemetery
8151 42nd Ave. North
New Hope, MN 55427
763-537-4184

Angela Warner Friend of the Foundation Award

In May 2003, the executive director of the Minnesota Chapter of the Cystic Fibrosis Foundation requested that I attend a luncheon with her and a Board member of the local chapter. During lunch, I was told about their proposal to rename the Chapter's annual award from the Friend of the Foundation Award to the *Angela Warner Friend of the Foundation Award*. The award is presented each year at the formal *Breath of Life Gala* to the person or family who made the greatest contribution that year to the success of the Chapter.

The request was an honor, but Linda and I had to weigh what we thought would be Angela's wishes. Angela did not want her life defined by a disease. Her life and everything about her was so much more than cystic fibrosis. Neither did Linda and I want our daughter's life after death to be identified solely with a chronic disease. However, Angie fought cystic fibrosis with courage, grace, and quiet discipline; she was an inspiration to others.

After careful deliberation, Linda and I decided to ensure with our own efforts that the renaming of the Foundation award and any other CF-related activities were only *part* of Angie's legacy, just as cystic fibrosis was only a part of her life, not the *whole* of her life! Linda and I accepted the invitation of the CF Foundation to honor Angie. As a result, each year at the *Breath of Life Gala*, Linda and I have the opportunity to present the award to the recipient.

The Twin Cities Breath of Life Gala has grown substantially in recent years to become one of the largest events of its kind in the nation, attracting as many as seven hundred attendees and raising more than one million dollars in an evening.

Few families stay active with cystic fibrosis foundations and causes after the loss of their loved ones to the disease. Linda and I understand these feelings. Staying involved, and being so vividly reminded of our child's suffering, is difficult. For this reason, we are selective about our commitments. But a cure must be found for this scourge on our children. A cure would relieve the pain and suffering of so many. A cure found may be bittersweet for those who have already lost their children, but we must *not* give up. *No* child should *ever* have to endure cystic fibrosis!

The Angela Brooke Warner Cystic Fibrosis Scholarship Endowment Fund

During the months and early years following Angie's death, I met individually with Dr. Warren Warwick and with Mary Jo McCracken. Mary Jo had been a pediatric pulmonary nurse practitioner/clinical nurse specialist for the University of Minnesota CF Center throughout Angie's entire life. Warren and Mary Jo were caring and supportive friends to Linda and me as we tried to process our grief and our feelings about Angie's medical care and the difficult decisions made during her last eighty-six days. Knowing of my desire to build the activities of the Angela Warner Foundation, they each independently shared with me the idea of providing a scholarship program to students with cystic fibrosis. Neither was aware of any similar program. After lengthy discussions with the University of Minnesota Foundation, Linda and I established an endowed scholarship at the University of Minnesota.

With advances in the care and treatment of individuals with cystic fibrosis in the past few decades, more adults with CF are living longer and more productive lives. Young adults with CF need a good education in order to attain the types of jobs that will support them and also provide comprehensive health insurance coverage, vacation and sick leave, short- and long-term disability insurance and a retirement plan.

With rising tuition costs, many college students with CF have jobs to help pay for their tuition and living expenses. A typical CF student in this position is tempted to skip therapy treatments, become sleep deprived, or compromise on their nutritional needs in order to meet their work and school commitments. The intent of the *Angela Brooke Warner CF Scholarship Endowment Fund* is to assist these young people in thriving as they balance school and work responsibilities with the demands of a chronic illness.

The University of Minnesota Foundation agreed to fully match any contribution Linda and I made to the endowment fund, therefore, doubling the scholarship for perpetuity. Linda and I first funded the endowment in 2005 and the first scholarship grant for $5,000 was presented. This annual scholarship continues to grow over time as our endowed contribution, and the matching endowed contribution, continues to grow. The Office of Disabilities at the University of Minnesota selects recipients.

The Angela Brooke Warner CF Scholarship Endowment Fund is an important and meaningful part of Angie's legacy of love.

Walks on the Beach with Angie: A Father's Story of Love

I put Angie's story in a book to help family and friends remember this special young lady and for people who never knew her to be inspired by her courageous and meaningful life.

The future of Angela's legacy of love has not been determined. Her spirit will provide the direction. So far, of the projects undertaken after Angie's death, this book has offered the greatest challenges and the deepest rewards. I wrote *Walks on the Beach with Angie: A Father's Story of Love* with only one critic in mind: *Angie.*

ACKNOWLEDGEMENTS

Don Warner says...

I am grateful for the honor I share with my wife, Linda, of being the proud parent of our courageous, loving and beautiful daughter, Angela. Angela blessed us by introducing us, directly or indirectly, to many remarkable people whom I thank for their parts in our lives.

To first acknowledge those closest to us, Linda and I have wonderful and loving families and friends who have been there for us during our hard times and our good times. They provide love, support, guidance, and gifts of laughter, peace, and comfort. There are not enough pages in this book to include each one by name, but they have our enduring gratitude.

I could not have told Angela's story without Linda's support. Writing this book was difficult for both of us, and she reviewed several versions of the manuscript and made many helpful suggestions. Thank you, my darling and beautiful wife.

I thank Josh Rasmusson, J.D. Eisenberg, Marcia Gallant, Pam Olson, Jackie Bordes, and Dick Johnson for their willingness to be interviewed and/or provide their unique perspectives to this book. I thank Amanda Roy, Brian Kuhl, and Mary Stevenson for their poetry, and Arthur Roy, Emily Schaefbauer, and Josh Rasmusson for allowing me to include their private correspondence.

During Angie's last eighty-six days, Linda and I were surrounded by loving family and friends, including Joan and Bill Sanford, Dick and Jeanne Johnson, Grant and Kathi Lindaman, J.D. Eisenberg, Josh Rasmusson, Linda's entire family, and all the frequent visitors and supporters.

Throughout those long emotional weeks, we had the privilege of meeting many exceptional people in the hospital "Family Room." In most cases, our lives crossed only briefly as together we encountered fear and despair, hope, and love. I thank each person with whom we spoke, prayed and spent time during those difficult days.

My profound thanks go to the ICU physician team at the University of Minnesota Medical Center and their professional and compassionate nursing staff. The surgical team, led by Dr. Greg Bielman, included Drs. Susan Seatter, Bruce Bennett, Ian Hasinov, Mia Evasovich, and Jeff Chippmann. Their care and efforts to save Angela, and cope with crisis after crisis, were truly heroic. Linda and I are also grateful for the love, support and spiritual guidance of two marvelous priests: Father Tim Power from Pax Christi Catholic Church and Father Steve LaCanne, the hospital priest. In the darkest of times, they offered friendship, comfort, and hope.

As children and young adults continue to battle cystic fibrosis, I remain grateful for the dedication of physicians such as Dr. Warren Warwick. I thank Warren for his lifelong work in caring for those with CF and striving for that elusive, yet achievable, cure. I specifically thank him for his loving care of Angela and his friendship with Linda and me. I am honored that he wrote the Foreword for this book.

I was able to speak with Frank Deford on several occasions while writing this book, and he gave me valuable encouragement, advice, and insights. I thank Frank also for his own book and his decades of service to the Cystic Fibrosis Foundation.

I thank those who helped Linda and me accomplish many wonderful things that are now a part of Angela's legacy of love: Jill Evenocheck and Molly Boyum at the Minnesota Chapter of the Cystic Fibrosis Foundation, John Cherek and Dave Kemp of The Catholic Cemeteries, and Steve Searl at the University of Minnesota Foundation.

Special thanks to my writing partner, Marly Cornell, who conducted interviews and transformed three year's worth of my revised manuscripts into an organized, coherent and final form. She often knew my thoughts and intentions before I voiced them. She was a blessing and a joy to work with always. Thank you, Marly.

Finally, every book becomes a collaboration of many talented people. In addition to Marly, I thank editor Pat Morris, publishing partners Corinne and Seal Dwyer, and my assistant Emily Schaefbauer. Thank you and all other contributors to this project for the journey we shared in creating *Walks on the Beach with Angie: A Father's Story of Love.*

Marly Cornell says...

I am privileged to have worked with Don Warner on his book about the life and loss of his lovely daughter, Angie, and the family's difficult struggle with cystic fibrosis. As a parent who also lost a daughter to a lifelong medical condition and disability, I did not expect our partnership to be such a joyful experience. However, Don remained an open and generous listener and collaborator, an astute critic and, at heart, a compassionate and devoted parent with a sincere wish to honor his child's life by helping others. I have thoroughly enjoyed the opportunity to know Angie through her father's eyes and those of her family and close friends. I now share the profound loss of a vibrant and precious young woman who lit up a room with her presence and dimmed the stars with her absence.

ABOUT THE AUTHOR

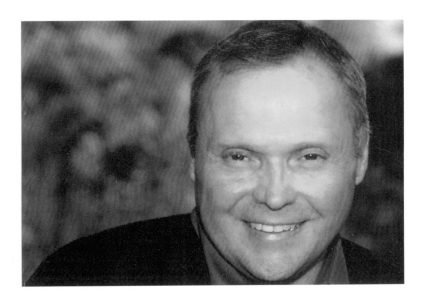

Don Warner is chief executive officer and chairman of the board of Wayzata, Minnesota-based New Era Financial Advisors, Inc., an investment advisory and financial planning firm he co-founded in 1982. He has worked closely with the Minnesota Chapter of the Cystic Fibrosis Foundation for many years and is a past board member of the University of Minnesota Pediatrics Foundation. Don and his wife, Linda, live in Eden Prairie, Minnesota, with their Maltese, Torrance.